Introduction to Research

A GUIDE FOR THE HEALTH SCIENCE PROFESSIONAL

Acquisitions Editor: Patti Cleary
Manuscript Editor: Patrick O'Kane
Indexer: Alexandra Weir
Art Director: Tracy Baldwin
Design Coordinator: Anne O'Donnell
Interior Designer: Adrianne Onderdonk Dudden
Cover Designer: Phoebe Darlington-Bush
Production Coordinator: Charlene Catlett Squibb
Printer/Binder: RR Donnelley & Sons, Inc.

6   5   4   3

Library of Congress Cataloging-in-Publication Data

Oyster, Carol K.
  Introduction to research.

  Bibliography: p.
  Includes index.
  1. Medicine—Research—Methodology.   I. Hanten, William P.
II. Llorens, Lela A.   III. Title. [DNLM: 1. Research—methods. W 20.5 O98i]
R850.O96 1987   610′.72   86-16111
ISBN 0-397-54626-2

To my daughter, Katherine
CKO

□□□□□□□□

ACKNOWLEDGMENTS

Sitting down and writing a textbook may well be the easiest part. This particular book would probably never have passed beyond the stage of an idea or a handwritten manuscript without the help and patience of some very special people:

the staff of the Computer Center at Goldey Beacom College, especially Elizabeth G. Davis, Sylvia Berta, and Patti Seay, who set up programs and answered a million dumb questions.

and Ms. Patti Cleary of J. B. Lippincott, who went well beyond her formal role as editor in consulting, consoling, and kibbitzing to become a real friend.

□□□□□□□□

INTRODUCTION

Research has a bad reputation. Many people think of research (and researchers) as dull, tedious, and plodding. We would like to think that just isn't so. To those of us involved in research, the entire process is somewhat akin to detective work or puzzle solving. We scan the environment for a question that needs to be answered, we employ our ingenuity and creativity to formulate questions that will result in evidence and clues that will help us make a deduction, and we evaluate the evidence to come up with a verdict. We hope that, as you read this text, you too will catch this flavor of mystery and excitement.

This is intended to be an introductory text. As such, it will merely introduce you to the major topics dealt with in research. For this reason, we have avoided deep theoretical discussions of the derivations and usefulness of various statistical procedures. In fact, we have for the most part avoided statistical formulas altogether.

Even if you expect never in your life to do research, as a clinician you will be expected to keep abreast of the new advances in your field. Who provides this new information? Researchers. As an informed consumer you should be familiar enough with the research process to determine when a study should be taken seriously. Particularly in a rapidly moving and developing area such as the health sciences, such knowledge is essential.

So, relax. This won't hurt a bit!

□□□□□□□□

CONTENTS

□□ 1 □□

Foundations of Health Science Research

Before we begin to consider the many questions involved with how to do research, it is important to stop and ask ourselves why we conduct research. This may seem a foolish and self-evident question to those readers who may have plans to join the research-associated division of their chosen profession. Most readers, however—indeed most who become health science practitioners—choose to enter into the service-providing division of nursing, occupational therapy, or physical therapy. If service providers in the health sciences are truly to call themselves professional, it is vital that they understand the basic principles of research so that they can directly aid the patients with whom they come in contact and indirectly aid the scientific advancement of their disciplines.

If an understanding of research is so important, why do so many practitioners shrink from studying it? There are probably several reasons, but it seems very likely that a general misunderstanding of the research process has created a certain mystique, which many researchers have done nothing to destroy. Researchers who have themselves been caught up in the excitement and mystery they see in the research process may be jealous of sharing the object of their passion or unable to see that others might require any explanation of its attraction.

But the process of research is a fundamental human behavior. As we look around us, the world's natural phenomena excite our curiosity: Why is the sky blue? What makes rain turn into snow? The world becomes a more secure place when questions can be answered, mysteries solved. To the extent that we ask questions about the world, and then seek to satisfy our curiosity with answers, we are all researchers.

Science has taken this apparently ubiquitous human need to solve problems and imposed a structure, a patterned approach to answering questions. Sciences advance as answers to old questions suggest new dilemmas. Facts and answers build upon themselves. Today's science is yesterday's magic.

Let's look at an everyday research process, applying the proper scientific terminology to each step. Upon awakening one morning you glance out your window, trying to decide what type of clothing would be most appropriate for the day. As it happens, the sky is cloudy. Your research question? ''Will it rain?'' Why do you care? Because it will directly affect your subsequent behavior in terms of your choice of clothing.

At this point you can make two plausible guesses—what researchers refer to as hypotheses. Either (1) it will rain, or (2) it will not rain. In order to choose between them, you must gather information (data) that will help you decide. In this case you might turn on the radio for a weather report or look for a weather forecast in the newspaper. Since there is no way for you to know for sure, you must draw a conclusion and make a guess as to which of your two hypotheses is likely to be correct. Having decided, you will dress accordingly and either take precautions or leave the umbrella at home. The weather during the day will provide you with feedback—you will know whether you made the correct choice. This feedback may influence your future behavior. If you trusted a particular newspaper's weather report and it was incorrect, you may be more hesitant about trusting that source of data in the future.

Of course, this is an extremely simplistic example. Scientific research can be (and generally is) much more complex. It may not matter much whether I choose to carry an umbrella if it doesn't rain, but what if I administer a medication or treatment to patients that is ineffective, or even harmful? How sure do I need to be before making a decision? The better my data, the more convinced I will be of the correctness of my decisions. Scientific control helps provide me with ''better'' data.

Researchers communicate their findings to their professional colleagues through written research reports. The discipline advances as new techniques are adopted. But how do you, as a practitioner, determine whether a new technique is useful, or even safe? In order to be a good consumer of research information, a practitioner must be able to understand the written research report and able to evaluate the quality of the research. It is to that end that the health sciences are increasingly requiring that future practitioners study research techniques as part of their professional training.

□ RESEARCH CONCEPTS APPLIED □
TO THE HEALTH SCIENCES

This book presents formal scientific research principles. The ideal, naturally, would be to employ perfect technique throughout every research project. This is not always (or even often) possible. The extent to which the rigid control required by the scientific method can be applied in practice depends on factors such as the subject matter of the discipline under study (e.g., much more control is possible when examining chemical reactions in a flask than when studying the effectiveness of an antibiotic *in vivo*).

By employing a composite index based on the amount of control possible, the directness with which the phenomena of research interest can be observed, and the length of time that formal research principles have been employed, it is possible to rank-order scientific disciplines. The "hard" sciences, such as chemistry and physics, allow for a very close adherence to the purest of research principles because very close control is possible with physical entities such as grams of sulphur, in part because of the stability and predictability of the elements and their interactions. In addition, research has been conducted for hundreds of years in these fields, thus allowing time for facts to accumulate and applications of principles to develop.

The social sciences, such as psychology and sociology, lag behind in the precision with which purest research principles may be employed. Human behavior is observable, but the individual variability and complexity of people makes control difficult. Ethical concerns limit the procedures to which human subjects may be subjected, which also may compromise the purity of research principles. Finally, formal research has only been an ideal in the social sciences for a relatively short period (since the early 1960s).

The health sciences have long been considered a subsidiary part of the art/science of medicine and have only recently (within approximately the last decade) begun to step forward as scientific disciplines in their own right. For this reason, at present there is relatively little systematic, scientific research available as the basis for further research. The phenomena of interest to researchers in the health sciences generally deal with medical events that are not directly observable and that involve essentially uncontrollable human subjects. Add to these difficulties the ethical constraints that dealing with human subjects entails, and it is hardly surprising that strict applications of pure research principles are seldom possible.

Given these constraints, why should a book on research principles for health science practitioners focus on principles that, in essence, are unattainably rigorous? The acceptance of a discipline as "scientific" depends upon adherence to these principles. As the health sciences evolve scientifically the possibilities for closer adherence will become greater. Knowledge of the principles of research allows researchers and consumers of research to recognize where compromises have been made and whether compromises are appropriate. Creativity and imagination on the part of researchers lead to designs that more closely approximate the ideal. It is the intent of this text to provide pure scientific research principles as an eventual goal for the health sciences, to point out situations in which their application may be especially problematic for health sciences research, and to suggest appropriate compromises.

The choice of the topic area and specific problem on which to conduct research is the most basic— and probably the most important— step in the research process. Research should expand the knowledge of an area; therefore, careful consideration should be given to this phase of the research. Choosing a problem that has already been extensively studied is a potentially expensive redundancy. On the other hand, choosing an appropriately unique problem that is poorly conceptualized and stated may result in the collection of data that either are not relevant to the question at hand, or are not collected in a form that makes statistical analysis possible. Since (as is discussed in Chapter 11) statistical decision-making is an important part of the research process, you might find yourself in the awkward and embarrassing position of having wasted your resources (time and money) collecting worthless information.

□ FINDING A PROBLEM □

Researchable problems in the health sciences can be chosen from a number of sources. There are essentially two types of research—basic and applied. Basic research seeks to uncover the underlying principles of phenomena. An example of basic research would be investigation into exactly what happens in the brain to result in the confusion of patients with Alzheimer's disease. Basic research in the health sciences is often within the realm of medical research conducted by physicians or PhDs in the basic medical sciences.

Applied research can be thought of as the logical extension of basic research in that it seeks practical uses for the findings of basic research by applying those principles in real-world or clinical settings. Thus, applied research might investigate which of two treatments is more effective in patients with Alzheimer's disease. Research in the health sciences is more likely to be of the effectiveness-testing, applied variety.

Clinical experience provides a wealth of potential research topics. Given that practitioners have the autonomy to choose among a variety of treatments, it would be most useful to know which treatment is most effective when applied to a particular condition.

But why bother with research? Certainly everyone knows what works and what doesn't, and speaking with other service-providers will give you that information. One reason is that individual practitioners may deal with a relatively small number of cases of a particular type, even over the span of a career. These cases are intermixed with many other types of cases. Memory is a remarkably unreliable phenomenon. A clinician may choose a favorite technique because it worked once, because everyone uses this technique (the force of tradition), because it is easier and more efficient, or because he or she is not aware of other treatments. The control and attention to objectivity of the research situation helps to reduce the number of uncontrolled alternatives and can help us to determine when treatment is indeed most effective.

Advances in medical technology also provide topics for research. When a new, untested treatment becomes available it is most important that before an automatic switch is made, the treatment be proven not merely effective, but more effective than traditional alternative treatments.

Reading through the literature (either textbooks or the journals in your discipline) can also stimulate research. A basic tenet of this text is that one should always question. Why are you told that Treatment A is more effective than Treatment B? Is any support cited? Why, in a particular research study on aphasia, did the author choose to conceptualize the variables in this particular way? What would happen if instead you were to reconceptualize and redefine the measures used? Would that change the results of the study? A single piece of research cannot answer all possible questions, and sometimes the researcher doesn't recognize an oversight or underlying assumption that affects the results until it is too late (the data are in). Clearly, the next step is to repeat (replicate) the study, correcting for these earlier problems or taking the next logical step.

Testing and expansion of theory is a basic role of research. Theories are developed through the findings of research and the expanded theory provides the questions for further study, in a circular pattern. The role of theory in the formulation of research studies is discussed in Chapter 2.

Now, you have an idea in which you're interested. At this stage you're usually asking a question such as: Is the level of performance achieved in a work adjustment group in a hospital setting predictive of work adjustment in a community setting outside the hospital? The next step is to move into the literature to discover whether others have explored this question and, if so, what they have found.

□ LOCATING SOURCES □

Researchers communicate their findings to their colleagues through journal articles, books, monographs, and conference proceedings. These written records are accessible to you in libraries. Libraries themselves provide many aids and services to help you find just those sources that will provide you with the information you need.

The card catalog is a file of cards listing all the publications in the library. In most cases, there are separate catalogs for books and periodicals. Each publication is represented in the catalog by several cards, which are filed alphabetically.

The author card is filed under the author's last name. If there are several collaborating authors, a card is filed for each one. Where there is no author for a particular work, the card is filed under the name of the society or association that prepared the publication.

The subject card lists the major topic area of the publication, such as occupational therapy, physical therapy, or nursing. Additional cards may appear under subheadings such as motor assessment scales, therapeutic exercise, or intensive care nursing. For biographies or autobiographies, the subject card is listed under the name of the subject of the book. The title card is listed under the title of the work with any preceding article dropped.

The types of card listings just mentioned are the ones found in most libraries. In some, another card, known as the analytical card, is also found. This card actually delves into the contents of a publication and provides listings for important names and issues within the text of the work. It may be thought of as a more in-depth subject card.

The card catalog is designed to help you locate the book you want. It does this by listing each book under several headings, which allows you to find the call number, which in turn tells you where this work is located in your particular library.

Two basic classification systems are used to locate books, the Dewey-Decimal system and the Library of Congress system. These are summarized in Table 1-1. As you can see, the major subject categories are quite broad in both systems.

Suppose you want a certain work and you can't find any listing for it under any of the categories listed in Table 1-1? That means your library doesn't contain this work. But do not despair—all is not lost. Many institutional libraries have a reciprocal arrangement with other libraries called interlibrary loan. In effect, your library borrows the book from another li-

TABLE 1-1 LIBRARY CLASSIFICATION SYSTEMS

Dewey Decimal System	*Library of Congress System*
000 General references, Periodicals, Cyclo- pedias, Biography	A General works
	B Philosophy, Religion
100 Philosophy, Psychology	C History
200 Religion	D World History
300 Social Sciences	EF American History
310 Statistics	G Geography
320 Political Science	H Social Sciences
330 Economics	I vacant
340 Law	J Political Science
350 Administration	K Law
360 Welfare Associations, and Institutions	L Education
370 Education (General)	LA History of Education
370.1 Theory and Philosophy of Education	LB Theory of Education
370.9 History of Education	LC Special forms and ap-
371 Teachers — Methods	plications
372 Elementary Education	LD U.S. Schools
373 Secondary Education	LE American Education
374 Adult Education	LF European Education
375 Curriculum	LG Asia, Africa, Oceania
376 Education of Women	LH School Periodicals
377 Religious, Ethical Education	LI vacant
378 Higher Education	LJ Fraternities, Sororities
379 Public Schools	LT Textbooks
379.14 School Law	M Music
379.15 Supervision and Control	N Fine Arts
380 Commerce, Communications	O vacant
390 Customs	P Language, Literature
400 Linguistics	Q Science
500 Pure Science	R Medicine
600 Applied Science	S Agriculture
700 Arts and Recreation	T Technology
800 Literature	U Military Science
900 History	V Naval Science
	W–Y vacant
	Z Library Science, Bibliog- raphy

brary so that you can then borrow it from your library. Complex? Not really. Your librarian will assist you in the process.

□ THE REFERENCE ROOM □

Perhaps in looking through the card catalog you found above the call number of a particular work the notation "Ref. Room." Not all books in any library are available for loan. Some, because they're rare or expensive or frequently accessed, are placed in the reference room. The reference room contains a number of useful aids to the would-be researcher.

One of the resources available in the reference room is the collection of reference books on references. Occasionally, you will only have sketchy information on a potentially useful article or book. These references will help you to obtain further information. One such reference is the volumes in *Books in Print*. All books still being printed appear in these volumes, which have listings for title, author, and subject.

Another potentially useful reference is *American Reference Books Annual*, published in Littleton, Colorado, by Libraries Unlimited since 1970. This volume, which annually provides reviews written by library specialists of reference works, is probably the most comprehensive guide to references.

If you need information about a journal you can turn to the *Standard Periodicals Directory*, published in New York biannually since 1964. Over 30,000 entries covering every type of periodical (except newspapers) are arranged under 200 classifications by subject. An alphabetical index is provided.

Journals are the most important resource for the literature review and search because they present the most recent information. In technologically advancing disciplines such as the health sciences, information contained in books becomes dated very quickly, partly because of the time involved in the publication process. Journals are usually bound by libraries into annual volumes and shelved in the library stacks. These volumes usually may not be removed from the library.

Since you are interested in a particular research question, one method of approach might be to determine which journals publish research pertaining to your topic, and then search through issues of each journal for relevant articles. This could become quite a tedious and time-consuming task.

Journals frequently provide abstracts (short summaries) of articles at the end of each issue. Although this helps shorten the time involved in your search, it would be even more useful if instead of having to search each issue of a journal you could have a collection of abstracts to search. There are several such collections in the reference room that you may find useful.

Excerpta Medica includes abstracts from over 5000 journals plus books and conference reports in the biomedical field. To facilitate your search, listings are divided into 42 sections with seven index sections. Once you have located an abstract that appears relevant to your topic of interest you can use the information in the listing to find the original article. *Psychological Abstracts* provides a similar collection of abstracts from journals covering psychology and the behavioral and social sciences and from selected nursing journals.

Abstracts provide a brief summary to help you determine whether the article is relevant to your interests. Less information is provided by the various indexes available in the reference room.

Index Medicus provides a comprehensive index to the world's medical literature. The index includes thousands of journals and is published monthly. There are both subject and author indices.

Research Quarterly is the research journal for the American Alliance for Health, Physical Education, and Recreation. This journal has provided ten-year indexes since 1930. The American Occupational Therapy Association has published an index of the *American Journal of Occupational Therapy* from the beginning of the journal to 1971.

Current Contents is a weekly booklet containing tables of contents from over 900 journals in the life sciences plus journals in the physical sciences, chemistry, the behavioral sciences, education, food and veterinary sciences, engineering and technology. It includes an author index complete with addresses so you can write to request reprints of articles of interest.

□ COMPUTER SEARCHES □

Technological advances have provided a very quick, comprehensive way to conduct a literature review and search—the computer or automated search. No knowledge of computers is necessary as the search is actually conducted by a librarian trained in the use of the various data bases available.

On-line computer terminals are linked to retrieval systems such as SDC/ORBIT, DATRIX II, and ERIC (Educational Resources Information Center). You complete a request for a search indicating the topic of interest, including any key words or phrases and the names of any important authors. You also provide any limits you wish to impose on the search (such as a request to search only the last five years of the literature). The librarian chooses the appropriate data base(s) and conducts the search.

You generally receive a hard copy of the listing of relevant references and a bill. Computer searches usually are not free. However, you must bear in mind how much more rapid and comprehensive than a manual search they may be.

A word of warning: Computer searches are only as useful as the initial information you provide to the librarian. Be sure to take the time to think of the key words that will exhaust your topic.

There are several data bases that are particularly relevant to the health sciences. These include MEDLARS and MEDLINE and SCISEARCH.

MEDLARS (Medical Literature Analysis and Retrieval System) includes *Index Medicus* from 1964, *Index to Dental Literature*, and the *International Nursing Index*. Over 1,800,000 citations to over 3,000 journals in the medical and health professions are included.

MEDLINE (MEDLARS on line) is a newer and faster system that was established in 1974. MEDLINE contains a smaller data base consisting of 1200 journals.

SCISEARCH corresponds to the Science Citation Index and contains all areas of science, including the biological areas. It also includes the Smithsonian Science Information Exchange data base, which contains reports and abstracts of research supported by 1300 government agencies and private organizations.

Now you have collected a group of references that appear to be relevant to your research question. Your next step is to collect and read the articles themselves. Some you will be able to discard immediately as not relevant. For those that seem relevant, pay attention to the reference section. Are there any references there that look as if they might be worth running down?

□ EVALUATING THE LITERATURE □

At this point in the process you have collected a number of published studies you believe to be relevant to your topic of interest. You have, therefore, an idea of how many other people have approached your problem in a systematic fashion and you know what they report having found. What you still need to determine is whether these articles will be useful to you in your research.

If you read that last sentence again, you may recognize the underlying assumption that all research is not created equal. Just because a study has cleared the hurdles and made it into print is no guarantee it is well-done research. Which leads to our first rule for evaluating the literature: Do not believe everything you read! Approach any written material (even this text) with a skeptical attitude and your critical facilities at the ready. Most authors do not deliberately set out to fool the public, but unfortunately the literature is full of well-intentioned mistakes.

How do you go about evaluating a study? In many respects that is what this entire text is about. Many of you probably will not conduct extensive research, but that is no reason you should not develop the expertise necessary to critically evaluate the research literature.

The objectives of this section are to provide you with a framework for analysis, to point out critical features, and to direct you to the later sections of the text that discuss these issues further. Most health science research reports are presented in a standard format consisting of sections headed Introduction, Methods (or Materials and Methods), Results, and Discussion. The following treatment of research papers will follow the same format.

Introduction

Within the introductory section of the paper, the author should cite the studies upon which this particular piece of research is based, and will state the reason for the research in terms of a researchable question or hypothesis.

Your first task is to consider the literature review. Do the studies cited appear relevant to the author's stated interest? Is it clear what these earlier authors found and what the relevance of their findings is to the question at hand? In other words, given this research as background, would you have been led to the author's hypotheses?

What about the hypotheses themselves? It should be clear to you from the introduction exactly what the study was investigating. The hypotheses should be explicitly stated (listing what is to be done) and outcome predictions should be made (listing expected findings). The predictions or expected findings should be clearly related to the earlier research cited. At the end of the introduction, therefore, you should be able to answer the following questions:

1. What other research has been published on this topic?
   a. What did these studies find?
   b. How is this relevant to the present topic?
2. What is the hypothesis of this study? What is to be researched?
   a. Is the hypothesis clearly and directly related to the previous research?
   b. Is the hypothesis stated in such a way that it is clear exactly what is to be done in the present study?
3. What results are expected for the present study?
   a. Can you determine why these particular predictions are being made?
   b. Are the predictions stated explicitly enough that you know exactly what evidence would be necessary to determine whether the predicted outcomes have occurred?

Chapter 2 of this text expands on these issues.

Methods

Having examined the theoretical underpinnings of the research, we move now to examine its structure. We have our questions and we want to be sure the design allows us to collect data that will answer them. Basically, we have three classes of research design: 1) experimental designs, 2) quasi-experimental designs, and 3) non-experimental designs. These vary

TABLE 1-2 QUESTIONS TO APPLY IN EVALUATING THE LITERATURE

Introduction
1. What other research has been published on this topic?
   a. What did these studies find?
   b. How is this relevant to the present topic?
2. What is the hypothesis of this study? What is to be researched?
   a. Is the hypothesis clearly and directly related to the previous research?
   b. Is the hypothesis stated in such a way that is clear exactly what is to be done in the present study?
3. What results are expected for the present study?
   a. Can you determine why these particular predictions are being made?
   b. Are the predictions stated explicitly enough that you know exactly what evidence would be necessary to determine whether the predicted outcomes have occurred?

Methods
1. What type of design was used for this study?
2. Why was this design the best choice given the hypothesis of the study?
3. Are there any practical or ethical constraints that led to the use of this design?
4. What is (are) the independent variables employed?
   a. Do(es) these variables embody the questions asked in the hypothesis?
5. Do the dependent measures employed flow from the hypothesis?
   a. Are these the best measures to answer the research problem?
   b. Are the variables clearly defined?
   c. Are there other, better ways this concept could have been measured?
6. Why were these particular subjects chosen for this research?
   a. Are these subjects suited for this study, or would some other group of subjects have been more appropriate?
   b. Where and how were these subjects recruited and/or convinced to participate in this study?

Results
1. What statistical procedures were employed?
   a. Are these tests appropriate for the research design employed?
   b. Are the results stated clearly? (Do you know which group or treatment was "best", or whether a single treatment was "effective"?)
   c. If a statement is made concerning "statistical significance" or "reliability", what significance level (alpha level) was employed?

Discussion
1. In terms of the research hypothesis, what did this study find?
   a. What questions does it answer (or provide evidence for)?
   b. What questions doesn't it answer?
2. What are the limitations of the study?
   a. What could/should have been done differently?
   b. What changes should be made for the next study in this line of research?
   c. Are there any concerns regarding application of results (generalizability)?

along two continua—control and what we can call "naturalness". Experimental designs provide us with the most control, thus leading to more certainty about the forces determining our results. However, this very control may create an artificial situation unlike that found in the real world. Since the ultimate goal of research is often to apply (generalize) our results to practical settings, such control may not really be desirable. It may also be the case that the very nature of our phenomenon of interest may severely limit either the number of subjects available for study or the kinds of experimental manipulations ethically allowable. For example, just because we are interested in examining the responses of brain-damaged patients in certain settings, we cannot deliberately create subjects by injuring people. All of these issues play a role in determining which research design should be employed for a particular study. Questions you should ask to evaluate research design include:

1. What type of design was used for this study?
2. Why was this design the best choice given the hypothesis of the study?
3. Are there any practical or ethical constraints that led to the use of this design?

Chapters 3 through 6 of this text expand on these questions.

Moving deeper into methodological considerations, we need to identify and evaluate the variables that the study employs. To step away from research for a moment for an analogy, once we've determined whether to use a novel, a play, or a poem to tell our story, we must concentrate on choosing the words that best convey our ideas.

There are two major categories of variables: independent and dependent variables. Independent variables represent categories of membership, either naturally occurring or artificially created by the researcher. These categories represent differences in the research phenomenon of interest. A comparison of the time it takes for male and female stroke victims to regain speech makes use of the natural categories of gender. Comparing the speed with which ultrasound and massage reduce muscle spasms involves assigning experimental subjects to treatment groups that represent levels of the independent variable "method of treatment."

Dependent variables are our data measures. We believe they are dependent for their size or amount on the category-membership (or level) of the independent measure—hence the name. In the examples given above, number of days to regain speech and reduction in muscle spasm were the dependent measures. We must be very careful to define both independent and dependent measures in concrete, measurable ways. Both the units of measure (days, steps taken, extent of limb mobility) and any criterion measures (regained speech defined as a useable vocabulary of a specific number of words) must be clearly defined.

As well as being clear, the variables must be chosen so that they answer the questions posed by the research hypothesis. They must measure the appropriate phenomena in the most appropriate fashion.

In reading the piece of research you are seeking to evaluate, can you answer these questions?

1. What are the independent variables employed?
   a. Do these variables embody the questions asked in the hypothesis?
   b. Are they clearly stated in concrete, measurable terms?
2. Do the dependent measures employed flow from the hypothesis?
   a. Are these the best measures to answer the research problem?
   b. Are the variables clearly defined?
   c. Are there other, better ways this concept could have been measured?

Chapter 2 expands on the concepts of variable definition, Chapters 7 through 9 concern design of dependent variables.

One final concern about structure pertains to the subjects on whom the research was conducted. We need to consider who these people (or animals) were, how they were chosen as subjects, how many subjects were employed, and how they were assigned to treatment condition (in the case of experimenter-created levels of independent variables). Ask yourself:

1. Why were these particular subjects chosen for this research?
   a. Are these subjects suited for this study, or would some other group of subjects have been more appropriate?
   b. Where and how were these subjects recruited and/or convinced to participate in this study?

Chapter 3 discusses issues involved with sampling procedures.

Results

Once the data are obtained, the researcher's next task is to determine (and communicate) the results of the study. This is done by use of descriptive and inferential statistical procedures that allow the researcher to summarize and describe the data (descriptive statistics) and to determine whether any apparent effects of treatment (or group differences) can be assumed to be related to category membership (level of independent variable) or appear to be due solely to chance factors.

Mathematical statisticians have developed numerous statistical procedures applicable to various types of research designs and data structures.

For the results of a study to be meaningful, the appropriate tests must be employed.

To evaluate the statistical (results) section of the study you are examining, you should determine the following:

1. What statistical procedures were employed?
   a. Are these tests appropriate for the research design employed?
   b. Are the results stated clearly? (Do you know which group or treatment was "best", or whether a single treatment was "effective"?)
   c. If a statement is made concerning "statistical significance" or "reliability", what significance level (alpha level) was employed?

Statistical issues are discussed in Chapters 10 through 13 of this text.

Discussion

The results section of a research report tells you what the data indicated. The final section—the discussion—should tell you what the results mean and how they fit into the larger context of research in this area. In other words, this section should tie up all the loose ends. It should also draw your attention to any author-identified limitations of the study. After reading the discussion you should be able to determine the following:

1. In terms of the research hypothesis, what did this study find?
   a. What questions does it answer (or provide evidence for)?
   b. What questions doesn't it answer?
2. What are the limitations of the study?
   a. What could/should have been done differently?
   b. What changes should be made for the next study in this line of research?
   c. Are there any concerns about application of results (generalizability)?
3. Do the results of this study raise any new questions in the area?

As you can see, only knowledge of the research process will allow you to become a critical consumer of the research literature. Having introduced the general research framework and the pivotal questions and issues at each stage of the process, let us begin in Chapter 2 to examine each step in further detail.

□ SUMMARY □

Problems on which to conduct health-science research can be chosen from a number of different sources, including clinical experience, advances in medical technology and treatment, and the literature of the discipline that reports the results of previous research.

The library provides a rich source for research problems in journals, books, monographs, and conference reports. Aids in locating specific articles or references include the card catalog, the Reference Room, and, most recently, on-line computer searches of various data bases.

Researchers must develop skills as informed consumers of the written literature. Skills must be developed in evaluating the quality and usefulness of particular references. The relevance of the article and research to the problem of interest, the design and procedures of the research study, the statistical analyses of obtained data, and the significance of results must all be subject to evaluation.

□ KEY TERMS □

basic research
applied research
replication

□□ 2 □□

Stating the Problem

At this point in the research process you have chosen a particular question that you would like to investigate and you have an idea of what others have done in the area. There are several further important steps to be taken before you can begin collecting data. First, you must formulate the problem in such a way as to address the question appropriately. In other words, your question must elicit the answers you seek. If you want to know what time it is, you don't ask someone about the weather. If you need to know exactly to the second what time it is, you will word your question accordingly. In this chapter we will move through a refining process that will allow you to take a global research question such as "How effective is TENS (transcutaneous electrical nerve stimulation)?" and mold it into a researchable hypothesis.

17

□ THE ROLE OF THEORY □

Earlier we discussed the reasons for conducting research and decided that the two primary reasons involve the broadening of knowledge in the health sciences and the movement to bring the health sciences into line with the more "scientific" disciplines. At this point we need to discuss for a moment the characteristics of the scientific approach and the role of research in the process.

According to Bunge (1967, p. 27), "The primary target of scientific research is, then, the advancement of knowledge." This supports our earlier contention. However, eventually something must be done with the potentially isolated pieces of information generated through the research process. The facts must be put together into related clusters that help somehow our understanding of some phenomenon. This is one role of scientific theory. Indeed, we find that

> data are meaningful and can be significant only in a theoretical context, and that the haphazard accumulation of data, or even of information-packaging generalizations, when unaccompanied by a theoretical processing capable of accounting for the former and of guiding research, is largely a waste of time. One cannot know whether a datum is significant until one is able to interpret it, and data interpretation requires theories. (Bunge, 1967, p. 382)

Developing, testing, and expanding theories is an important aspect of science. In fact, Kerlinger (1965, p. 110) goes so far as to state that "the basic aim of science is theory." In our consideration of theory we will examine goals and purposes of theory, the process of theory construction, and the evaluation of theories.

The Goals of Theory

Scientific theories serve many purposes and several authors have compiled lists of these goals. Bunge (1967), in a particularly exhaustive effort, has listed the following six aims: (1) to systematize knowledge, (2) to explain facts, (3) to increase knowledge, (4) to enhance the testability of hypotheses, (5) to guide research, and (6) to offer a map of a chunk of reality.

Systematizing knowledge is the clustering process referred to above. Facts are collected that are associated with a particular phenomenon. Then, through the process of inductive and deductive reasoning, logical relationships are established. These speculative relationships, or hypotheses, form the basis for research. They help to explain the facts that have been generated through research and also help to generate further research themselves.

Once systems of facts have been pieced together they can serve as the basis for prediction as well as explanation. If we believe event *A* is related to the subsequent occurrence of event *B* and if we can detect or cause event *A*, then when event *A* occurs we can make a prediction about the outcome, which will then provide a test of our hypothesis.

Theories serve as a guide to research in three separate ways: "by posing or reformulating fruitful problems"; "by suggesting the gathering of new data which would be unthinkable without the theory"; and "by suggesting entire new lines of investigation" (Bunge, 1967, p. 383). By providing unique combinations of existing information, theories serve to suggest both tests of the hypothesized relationships and further novel approaches. Again, we are confronted with the circular relationship between research and theory wherein research provides new material for theorizing, which results in hypotheses to be tested through further research, and so on.

The final goal of theory (offering a map of reality) may appear relatively trivial on first examination, but it is actually extremely important. The first goals were related to the activity of science—explanation, prediction, and research. This final goal in contrast appears mundane and uncreative. Mapping and cataloging, however, provide a clear vision of the limits of our knowledge and thinking. Often it is in listing what we know that the gaps and limits become evident. In an expanding field, providing a map of the frontiers of knowledge becomes one of the most important functions of theory.

Theory Construction

There exist no rules for the construction of theories, although the process of theory construction may be traced from the pretheoretical stage of a discipline to the stage of formal theories. In the beginning a discipline consists of the ordinary knowledge and common-sense beliefs of practitioners. It is within this context that early theory construction takes place. These earliest efforts are a most difficult task. Once facts have been sorted and logically consistent relationships hypothesized, the theory becomes part of the context in which later theorizing takes place. A barrier to early theory building is that in the early stages of a discipline's evolution, the conceptual thinking is rather vague. As theories are put forward, the concepts become more clearly defined and thus more easily utilized.

Early theories, then, consist primarily of statements of logically consistent relationships between known facts. Once a theory has been created, it begins, with the aid of research findings, to evolve an increasingly precise, formal structure. The older sciences consist of highly formal theories that state nonempirical hypotheses in the formal language of mathematics, such as Einstein's famous statement of the equivalence of mass and energy, $E = mc^2$. Clearly, such precision requires quite a bit of information beyond that possessed by early theorists—information provided by research.

The foregoing discussion makes it sound as though theory construction consists merely in fitting the jig-saw puzzle pieces provided by research into some intuitively appealing whole. In fact, however, theory construction is as difficult and creative an act as painting a picture or writing a song. A theory is not a mere summary of data. Data provide the inspiration and eventually data help to point out the strengths and weaknesses of the theory—these are the endpoints of the process. The actual theory is an alchemist's brew consisting of the knowledge and technique available in the discipline at the time, existing theories, and the training, background, and biases of the theorist. Because the art of creation is essentially undefinable, the best that can be done to guide the process is to establish the goals and purposes that a theory should have (as above) and to establish criteria with which to evaluate the finished product. The gap between intention and evaluation is filled with inductive and deductive logical reasoning—the magic of theory construction.

Theory Evaluation

Essentially two types of criteria are used in the evaluation of a theory (Roy and Roberts, 1981). The first type examines the quality of logical thinking and concepts in the theory. The theoretical relationships and hypotheses must conform to the formal rules of logic and must be internally consistent with one another. The basic concepts must be definable and clear.

The second type of criteria used to evaluate a theory inspects more structural aspects of the theory. The first consideration is the level of specificity of the theory. A completely concrete catalogue of facts would not qualify as a good theory. A theory should be specific enough to suggest tests of hypotheses and at the same time contain abstract concepts. Without the abstract quality, the theory cannot hope to fulfill the heuristic role of good theory. For a theory to be valuable, it is not enough for it just to explain the particular set of facts that led to its introduction; it must also be capable of explaining other phenomena, predicting other effects, or generating further hypotheses.

A second important concern is the clarity of the theory. No matter how elegant the concepts or unique the hypothesized relationships, unless the scientific community can understand and therefore apply the concepts, the theory is useless. Clarity is particularly difficult to achieve in the early phases of a discipline's theory building. Poorly defined concepts are extremely difficult to communicate clearly. Thus, the level of evolution of the discipline as well as the clerical skill of the theorist will influence the level of clarity achieved.

The principle of parsimony is an important consideration in the evaluation of a theory. Parsimony is essentially the level of succinctness of the theory. In other words, a theory that can be clearly delineated in one hundred words is more desirable than a similar theory that requires one thousand words for its exposition. Parsimony and clarity are closely interrelated. The theory must be explained completely enough to be clear and at the same time be economical enough with explanation to be concise.

A final criterion for the evaluation of a theory (and one that is extremely important for research) is that the theory be operational. This means "it must be translatable into observable terms that can be measured" (Roy and Roberts, 1981, p. 15). Research seeking to test hypotheses is simply not possible unless the researcher has some idea, shared by the scientific community, of the definition of terms. In the behavioral sciences, particularly psychology, research has often been hindered by the lack of a clear definition of such terms as "anxiety" or "mental health." Without a shared and precise understanding of the meaning of concepts, researchers may adopt idiosyncratic definitions and thus, in effect, be examining different phenomena under the same label.

By now the extent of the entanglement between theory and research should be clear. It is virtually impossible to consider one without invoking the specter of the other. This is entirely appropriate, since both are essential to the development of a scientific discipline. But theory is not the end-all for science. Theory is but one step in the model of scientific knowledge to be presented below. Placing theory in the perspective of this model will allow us to consider the evolutionary status of the various health-science disciplines.

□ A MODEL OF SCIENTIFIC DEVELOPMENT □

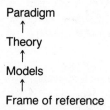

As can be seen from the model presented above, the earliest, lowest level aspect of scientific development pertains to the scientist's frame of reference. Essentially, the frame of reference can be thought of as the scientist's value system. Our models of thought and even our perceptions of the world are largely determined by the biases introduced by our value systems. Because the process is essentially out of consciousness, even the most objective scientist has difficulty escaping from these influences. The frame of reference is represented as the first step in the model because of its influence on the second step, the development and use of models. The level of the frame of reference is the most basic influence on the data the researcher chooses to gather. An example of different frames of reference might be seen in the different definitions of "improvement" employed by two health science practitioners in evaluating a stroke patient. One might define "improvement" as an increase in mobility while the other might define it as an increase in morale. Because of these differing definitions, the clinicians would be focusing on different aspects of the patient in examining the phenomenon they both described as "improvement."

Models are the next evolutionary step in the scientific process. Here facts and ideas are organized into symbolic representations of an idea or object. Within a discipline many models for specific situations may be generated without any attempt being made to interrelate the models. Often, the use of models in a discipline marks the turning point from a pretheoretical stage to the more "scientific" theoretical level. An example of a model would be a physical representation of the solar system using various sizes of spheres to represent the planets placed in such a way as to reflect their various distances from the sun. According to Reed (1984), "Models may describe, generate ideas, suggest explanations, interpretations or methodologies but do not meet the criteria of a theory" (p. 7). The influence of the frame of reference is felt through its determination of the philosophy and biases the scientist will bring to bear when determining which aspects to include in the model.

We have spoken a great deal about theory but never defined the term precisely. To borrow from Kerlinger (1965), a theory is "a set of interrelated constructs (concepts), definitions and propositions (assumptions) that present a systematic view of phenomena by specifying relations among variables, with the purpose of explaining and predicting the phenomena" (p. 11). The characteristics of explanation and prediction are the criteria Reed spoke of that differentiate a model from a theory. Roy and Roberts (1981) further delineate the differences between models and theories:

> As models describe their concepts, they tend to be general and overriding. The vagueness of the related terms of a model makes it difficult for them to be submitted to empirical testing. Theories, on the other hand, which can arise out of models, tend to deal with more specific phenomena within the models. Their terminology is more precise and concepts are defined in a way that they can be empirically tested. (p. 23).

In disciplines at this evolutionary level there may often be competing theories to explain specific phenomena, none of which is recognized as more acceptable than any other. For some people, for example, the conflict between the theory of evolution and the creation theory of human development can be a conflict between two equally possible explanations for an observed set of facts.

The final, most highly evolved stage in the development of a discipline is the paradigm. The paradigm is more comprehensive in that it may include several theories in a systematic, organized view of a subject. Generally only the older sciences, such as physics, have reached the stage of the paradigm and even here there are occasional (usually dramatic) shifts, as occurred when relativity theory replaced the older Newtonian physics. The paradigmatic level is characterized by general agreement within the discipline as to the reigning or "correct" world view.

The health sciences all exist at relatively low levels of development. Probably the most evolved discipline is nursing, which has developed both models such as the Roy Adaptation Model of nursing and theories such as the theory by Roy and McLeod (Roy and Roberts, 1981) of Adaptive Modes. Generally, however, there are many more models than theories in nursing. Physical therapy and occupational therapy both appear to reside primarily at the level of the model. Both disciplines, however, (as evidenced in part by the existence of this text) have stated an intention to focus more attention on research and the development of theory.

□ RESEARCH TERMINOLOGY □

Having discussed the importance of theory to science and research, we turn now to a consideration and definition of the components of theory. Use of these concepts will allow us to restate our theoretical research question in the precise way necessary to conduct acceptable research. We will begin with a consideration of the most elementary research component—the variable—and build to the definition and statement of hypotheses.

Variables

Variables are the basics of research. A variable is a measure whose value is not fixed and is therefore free to vary. Examples of variables are life satisfaction, vestibular function, and joint range of motion. Variables represent the phenomena of interest in a discipline.

Several types of variables are essential to the research process. Here we will discuss three: independent variables, dependent variables, and intervening variables.

Independent variables are the phenomena of interest in the research process. If we were comparing the efficacy of two modes of treatment for arthritis, we would be considering the independent variable Treatment

Type. We would refer to the two specific treatments as the two levels of our independent variable. In testing the effective dosage level of a medication we might try 1 ml, 5 ml, 10 ml, and 50 ml, thus obtaining four levels of the independent variable Amount of Medication. The categories of independent variables may be created by the researcher, as in the cases above, in which the researcher assigns a subject to a type of treatment or a dosage level. This type of artifically created or manipulated category is also known as an *active variable*.

It is often the case that the independent variable of interest cannot be assigned or manipulated by the researcher. If the researcher is interested in the effects of age on the response to medication, the levels of the variable are nonmanipulable demographic characteristics. Another naturally occurring category of interest to researchers is gender. This type of variable is also known as an *attribute variable*.

The independent variable may be loosely considered as the cause in the research problem. Manipulations of the independent variable are expected to create differences between groups on some outcome measure or dependent variable. We manipulate the dosage of drug to see what effect the various levels have on the clinical problem. Scores or measures on the dependent variable are thought to depend on the treatment, hence the name. In the same way that the independent variable may be thought of as the cause, the dependent measure of interest may be thought of as the effect. As long as the variable is conceptualized in a measurable form, almost any phenomenon of interest may be employed as either an independent or a dependent variable.

A special case of the dependent variable is known as the *criterion variable*, which Polit and Hungler (1982) describe as follows: "In studies that analyze the consequences of a treatment, therapy, or some other type of intervention, it is usually necessary to establish criteria against which the success of the intervention can be assessed" (p. 39). The criterion variable thus serves as a benchmark. All criterion variables are dependent variables and represent a special subset of this type of variable.

In some cases a direct causal relationship may not exist between independent and dependent measures in a study. The independent measure may affect an unmeasured factor that creates the changes in the dependent measure. Such a variable is known as an *intervening* or "nuisance" *variable*. For example, a researcher might institute classes in makeup and hair care for women who are institutionalized for clinical depression in the hopes of diminishing depressive symptoms. Probably improved appearance has some effect in improving self-concept, which in turn may reduce symptoms. Self-concept would be the intervening variable in this case. In this example the intervening variable could be (and probably should be) measured. It is often the case, however, that such variables cannot be controlled or measured directly. It is important in any case for the researcher to consider the possibility of the existence of one or more intervening variables in a proposed study and to control for or quantify such variables. Left unmeasured they may provide plausible alternative explanations for experimental results.

Defining Variables

Once a researcher has identified the variables of interest, he or she must take great care in defining and quantifying variables. It is unfortunately too common for researchers to spend insufficient time and thought on this step, which results in the collection of data that cannot be analyzed or interpreted. Certain statistical techniques are only appropriate when the data of the dependent variable are in a very specific format. (Of course, you can still apply a test to data based on an improper measurement scale. Your results, however, are useless. As an old computer phrase has it, "Garbage in, garbage out.")

Levels of the independent measure represent categories such as males vs. females, or TENS vs. ultrasound. The most important considerations in conceptualizing levels of the independent variable are that the levels must be mutually exclusive—that is, subjects cannot be classified at more than one level—and that the levels must cover the entire range of the phenomenon of interest. The number of levels of the independent variable has a bearing on the statistical techniques that may be employed.

An independent variable, for example, might be splint type in a comparison of the effects of several types of hand splints on hand-arm posture in hemiplegic children, or it could be the differences in expectations for improvement among stroke patients aged 30-39, 50-59, and 70-79. In the first example the independent variable is a discrete variable. The classes represent totally separate entities. A patient is wearing splint type A, B, or C. There is no B 1/2. Measurement of category is quite precise for this type of variable. Other discrete variables might be patient gender, patient diagnosis, or eye color.

Age, on the other hand, represents a continuous measure. It is not possible with continuous measures ever to be precisely accurate. If I state a patient's age as 36 years, 3 months, 21 days, 14 hours, I can still break the measure down into smaller units. If we wish to employ a continuous measure as an independent variable we must arbitrarily determine the boundaries between classes.

Continuous measures may also be employed as dependent measures. If we measure hand grip strength or range of motion we must recognize (at least on a theoretical level) that we have chosen a level of accuracy of measurement that could theoretically be improved.

Measurement Scales

There are four types of measurement scales that can be employed for dependent measures: (1) nominal, (2) ordinal, (3) interval, and (4) ratio. These will be presented in order of increasing complexity and statistical utility.

Nominal data are essentially qualitative data. Whenever we divide responses into categories we are using nominal data. If we were to measure the relative adoption of various forms of hand prosthesis, individuals would fall into a category based on their prosthetic device. Each element or individual in each category is equivalent to every other element. A child's prosthesis is categorized in precisely the same way as an adult's. For other studies, categories might include male or female or in-patient or out-patient. Once our data are sorted into categories, we count the number of elements in each. Because we do not have measurements (only counts) we are severely limited as to the statistical techniques that can be applied to data of this sort. It is better whenever possible to conceptualize your study so as to employ one of the mathematically more complex forms of measurement scale.

Ordinal data consist of rankings of measures. We use ordinal measures when ranking the order of finish in a race or (in the example above) ranking the order of popularity of prosthetic devices. Here we at least have a number associated with a measure rather than a category label. But mathematically, ordinal data are not much better than nominal data. Although we know the order of finish, we have no information about the intervals between finishers. In a marathon race the first-place finisher may come in minutes before the second-place finisher who comes in only seconds ahead of the person in third place. We can't say first is twice as fast as second. We don't have the kind of information we would need to make that statement. Ordinal data are very limited as to the statistics that can appropriately be applied, which severely limits our ability to draw conclusions from our data.

Interval scales are measurement scales in which there are equal intervals between the units of measure. There is, however, no absolute zero point. The Celsius temperature scale is a good example. Although there is a measure of 0° this does not mean the absence of heat. The 0° point was arbitrarily set at the point at which water freezes. So although it is true that the same amount of heat is necessary to raise the temperature from 4° to 5° as from 110° to 111°, we cannot say that 100° is twice as hot as 50°.

Ratio scales possess the qualities of interval scales (equal intervals between units) and also have a genuine zero point. If we are speaking of days since a patient sustained an injury, it is entirely possible to have a score of 0 (meaning the injury occurred today). We can also say someone injured 4 days ago has been injured twice as long as someone injured 2 days ago. Most statistical techniques require or can be applied to ratio measures.

Operational Definitions

The researcher must exercise great care not only in quantifying variables but also in precisely defining what is intended by the variable. In concrete cases such as patient age or degrees of limb mobility, the requisite precision is inherent in the measure. Often, such precise, concise measures are the goal of variable definition. But seldom are such precise definitions the intuitively satisfying goal of research. We tend rather to ask our questions in terms such as "Will Treatment A be effective with patients?" Here our independent variable is Treatment A, our dependent variable is "effectiveness," and we have a potential intervening variable—patient type.

In order to improve the exactness of these variables we must define the constructs involved. To do so we make use of operational definitions. An operational definition is the "delineation of the procedures and tools required to make the observations or measurements" (Polit and Hungler, 1983, p. 36). Although this definition is more generally applied in reference to dependent variables, it is also appropriate for independent variables. To elaborate on our example, Treatment A would be defined as the operations performed by the researchers on the patient. Effectiveness would have to be defined concretely in terms of some physical measure such as increase in mobility (in degrees of mobility) or decrease in pain experienced (as defined by decrease in requests for pain medication or grams of pain medication required per day, or increase in length of time between requests for medication). The units of measure are specified to force researchers to focus their thoughts and to allow other researchers to replicate the study. If I were simply to report that Treatment A "makes patients feel better," no one would know what I meant. If I specify the measures, they know precisely.

In our example the patient was identified as a potential intervening variable. Treatment A might prove wonderfully "effective" (using whatever measure the researcher has specified) for patients in some diagnostic categories, and useless or harmful to patients in other categories. Operationally defining patient here would involve narrowing (or at least specifying) the focus of our sample.

Conceptual Definitions

The researcher must also take care to define conceptual terminology that is used in stating the research question to avoid ambiguity. A conceptual definition may be secured from the dictionary or the professional literature, or it may be defined by the author. All terms that would not be considered to be generally well understood require definition.

Hypotheses

We have taken our global research question, identified the variables of interest, and operationally defined the variables. We are ready now to state our research hypotheses. The hypothesis is the relationship between the measures we will test experimentally. As such we no longer ask questions, we make a statement about what we believe about the relationship between the variables.

Two types of hypotheses are employed in research studies: experimental hypotheses and statistical hypotheses. The experimental hypothesis is our belief about the relationship between the variables; for example, ultrasound is more effective than TENS in decreasing muscle spasm. (We would, of course, go on to operationally define our measure of muscle spasm.) This is known as a directional hypothesis. We are willing to guess what effect our independent variable (treatment type) will have on our dependent variable. In medically oriented research we will often employ directional hypotheses, since our goal is to increase patient well-being. We have two directions of hypotheses, of course. Our dependent measures might involve increased self-esteem or expectations for recovery or reduced pain and increased mobility.

Sometimes—particularly in the early stages of a line of research—we will not be able (or willing) to guess the direction of an effect, but we want to test whether an effect exists. Such a nondirectional hypothesis might be stated: "Disabled Vietnam veterans and disabled Korean veterans will respond differently to group therapy." We anticipate some effect; we're just not sure what the effect will be.

Regardless of our experimental hypotheses, our research never assesses the hypothesis directly. All assessment is done statistically through direct testing of a statistical hypothesis known as the null hypothesis (H_0). At the end of a study we have a set of data that we hope will address our hypothesis and match our predictions. If we find our groups to be different at the end of the study, there could be a number of reasons for the differences. Maybe they were different to start with. Maybe our measures are off. And maybe our treatment was effective. We try to control for as many alternative explanations as possible by paying close attention to the issues of validity, reliability, and sampling. But we never really know the source of an apparent effect. What we test statistically is the size of the effect. The null hypothesis states that there really was no effect of our treatment and any apparent differences happened purely by chance.

Let's take a simple, concrete example. I show you a coin and tell you that through some exceptional mental powers I can make the coin come up heads when tossed. I toss the coin and it comes up heads. Are you impressed? I hope not. Why? Because a fair coin will come up heads 50% of the time. The event is very likely to occur by chance. Suppose I toss the coin nine more times and it comes up heads every time.

Now you should wonder. (After checking to see if it's a fair coin!) Why? Because the probability that you will hit ten heads in a row is approximately .001. If we sat around tossing coins in sets of ten repetitions, only in one out of a thousand such sets of throws would we expect to see ten heads. So either I'm incredibly lucky, or maybe I *can* control that coin. But it could happen by chance. The null hypothesis tests the mathematical probability that the results we obtain for our study could have happened by chance by measuring the probability of such an outcome if there really was no effect (or, in our example, if I really don't have control of the coin).

We state our null hypothesis (H_0) and our experimental hypothesis (H_a) so that they are mutually exclusive (e.g. H_0: Treatment A has no effect, and H_a: Treatment A reduces muscle tremor). We then directly assess the null hypothesis statistically. If my effect (as measured by a large difference either between groups or between pre- and post-treatment evaluation of patients) has a very low probability of occurring by chance I reject the statement that there is no effect. Since the alternative situation is the existence of an effect, I accept my experimental hypothesis.

If my results were very possibly the result of chance factors I fail to reject the null hypothesis. I *never* accept the null hypothesis. Why? Because the nonexistence of an effect is only one of a number of possible explanations for my results. Maybe my design was inappropriate. Maybe my treatment was not administered properly. Maybe my statistical test wasn't sensitive enough to perceive the effect. Or maybe my treatment didn't work. Since I can't distinguish between the reasons, I must fail to reject the null hypothesis. (This is a superficial discussion of an extremely important topic, which will be explored in depth in Chapter 11.)

Stating Your Hypothesis

A well-stated hypothesis (or hypotheses) is the essential basis for good research. The hypothesis is the basis upon which everything else rests. If the variables are not clearly defined and the hypothesized relationships between them clearly indicated, the research cannot hope to make any meaningful statement. A good hypothesis in turn rests on clearly delineated constructs and precise operational definitions of variables.

Three criteria are useful in evaluating a research hypothesis. The first is clarity. Since the hypothesis is a statement of relationship between variables, it should be very clear exactly what relationship the experiment is predicting. In the case of a complex phenomenon, it is perfectly acceptable to break the experiment down into several hypotheses. This is far more desirable than attempting to test one hugely complex, unclear hypothesis.

The second criterion is concreteness. This rests firmly upon the variables employed and on the level of specificity the researcher indicates for the relationship. Abstract concepts are not appropriate at this stage. Any abstract concepts should have been concretized through the use of operational definitions.

The final criterion is testability. It is essential that the hypothesis can be operationally tested or the research comes to a screeching halt. Think of the hypothesis as the road map indicating a route. The well-written hypothesis suggests the best way (or ways) of testing. Usually a clear, concrete statement of the relationship between two operationally defined variables will meet this criterion of testability.

A very important step has been taken in the research process. We began this chapter with a general question and finished with our variables defined and stated in a testable hypothesis. The next step in the process involves designing a study to test our hypotheses. Designs will be discussed in Chapters 4 through 6. Chapter 3 will discuss theoretical research issues that underlie all of the various designs.

□ SUMMARY □

The conduct of research is a step in the broadening of knowledge and in contributing to the scientific significance of the health-science disciplines. Theory creation is the process through which knowledge is systematized and organized to allow scientists to determine the areas in which knowledge exists and the areas in which further inquiry is needed. Theories are a step on a continuum of scientific development and organization that ranges from at the most basic level, the frame of reference through model and theory development to the overarching paradigm, which represents a systematic organization of theories into a coherent view of a discipline.

The basic questions addressed in research are known as hypotheses. Hypotheses consist of statements of the relationships between variables to be tested through research. Variables must be defined through concrete operational definitions and may be of several types: independent variables to be manipulated or measured by the investigator, dependent or outcome measures, and intervening or nuisance variables.

The types of data to be collected in research represent different types of measures. Nominal data consist of categories of objects or phenomena. Ordinal data represent rank orderings of measures. Interval measures are characterized by equal intervals between measurement points and the lack of a true zero point. Ratio measures possess equal intervals and a true zero point, thus rendering this type of data appropriate for a wide range of statistical procedures.

The well-designed research study consists of at least two hypotheses, the null hypothesis to be tested statistically and the alternative or experimental hypothesis. The thoughtfully stated hypothesis clearly suggests the optimal data format, collection procedures, and analyses for the research study.

□ KEY TERMS □

theory
paradigm
model
frame of reference
variable
independent variable
dependent variable
intervening variable
criterion variable
active independent variable
attribute independent variable

discrete variable
continuous variable
nominal scale
ordinal scale
interval scale
ratio scale
operational definition
hypothesis
experimental hypothesis
null hypothesis

□□ 3 □□
Basic Concepts: Validity, Reliability, and Sampling

- □ *Validity*
- □ *Threats to Validity*
  - □ *Statistical Conclusion Threats*
  - □ *Threats to Internal Validity*
  - □ *Threats to Construct Validity*
  - □ *External Validity*
- □ *Reliability*
  - □ *Instrument Reliability*
  - □ *Standardization of the Treatment of Subjects*
  - □ *Stability of Obtained Results*
- □ *Sampling*
  - □ *Probability Sampling*
  - □ *Nonprobability Sampling*
  - □ *Sample Size*
  - □ *Assignment of Subjects*

Once we have formulated our hypotheses, the next step in the research process is to design the study we will use to test them. Before we actually begin to conceptualize the structure of our design, there are a number of basic concepts to be considered. This chapter will discuss the experimental issues of validity, reliability, and sampling procedures.

□ VALIDITY □

In common usage we apply the adjective "valid" when something is perceived as being accurate or true. Dictionaries define the term as meaning "well supported by fact." In research design the term validity has several specialized applications.

Classically in the literature of research design the concept of validity has been dichotomized into internal and external validity (Campbell & Stanley, 1963). Internal validity refers to the relationship between the variables within the study. For a study to be internally valid, the variables must be logically consistent and represent a testable causal relationship. External validity refers to the extent to which the results of the study can be applied to other similar situations in the world—the extent to which the results can be generalized.

Cook and Campbell (1979) have broadened the concept of validity by introducing two additional categories. The following discussion of validity will draw heavily on the concepts presented in their work. The first category of validity was labeled Statistical Conclusion Validity. In evaluating the data of a study, statistical techniques assess the extent of covariation (variability shared) between the variables. The choice of statistical tests and their application determine the interpretation of the relationship between the variables. Incorrect uses of statistics, then, should be avoided because they can introduce sources of invalidity (i.e., misinterpretations) into the study's conclusions.

The second category of validity is Internal Validity. Once covariation between the variables has been determined, the next question is the extent and direction of causality between the variables. If a study examines variables A and B, there are at least three possible causal relations: (1) Variable A could cause variation in Variable B; (2) Variable B could cause the variation in Variable A; or (3) some unknown and/or unmeasured Variable C could be responsible for the variation in both Variables A and B. An internally valid study seeks to clarify the direction of the relationship.

The third category, Construct Validity of Putative Causes and Effects, was introduced by Cook and Campbell to deal with issues involving the theoretical constructs of the study. A construct is a theoretical concept to which a label has been applied (such as "anxiety" or "health") which is then dealt with as an entity. The concern of this type of validity is with the clarity of definition of the constructs involved in the study. It must be precisely clear what is being described when we speak of a construct such as health so that other researchers will understand and label the same phenomenon in the same manner.

Construct definition also involves reifying and narrowing a construct in the independent variable of a study to a level of clarity such that the cause of the change in the dependent variable is apparent. The dependent variable also must be formulated with this level of clarity: It is necessary to determine what aspect of the construct has been changed. Both of these requirements are facilitated by the use of operational definitions, as discussed in Chapter 2.

To assist in the explanation of construct validity as applied in this context, let us turn to a classic example from the health sciences. When a new medication is developed, controlled testing is, of course, necessary to determine the drug's effectiveness. Let us say that a new painkiller has been developed. We give this medication in capsule form to persons suffering pain and ask them to report on the effects. We find, much to our delight, that everyone is reporting relief from, or at least reduction in, pain. Is our drug effective? Maybe. Very possibly not. There are a number of rival explanations that are equally plausible.

Patients who receive medication for pain have the entirely appropriate expectation that the drug is intended to reduce (and not increase) their discomfort. Psychological research (Orne, 1969) has clearly demonstrated that expectations can become self-fulfilling prophecies. Thus our first alternative explanation is based on patients' expectations. In any medical setting this possible explanation is unavoidable.

If expectations were enough, physicians or nurses would need to do no more than tell patients to feel better. Sometimes, in fact (as in faith healing and folk medicine) this works. More often it is the ingesting of the substance that is believed to be helpful that produces the necessary mental set, which gives us a second possible explanation for our results—taking the capsule itself.

To circumvent this difficulty, pharmaceutical firms routinely make use of experimental techniques to clarify the actual cause of any change in the patient's condition. The most common is the use of a placebo. Some subjects are given the actual medication (in this case, our painkiller) and others are administered an inert substance in exactly the same manner (identical capsules or injections) and led to believe they are receiving medication. If only those patients receiving the actual medication experience a change, identifying the substance as the cause is much more easily defensible.

In checking for construct validity of putative causes and effects, Cook and Campbell identify four major areas to be considered. The first involves ascertaining the extent to which the "putative cause," or independent variable, has actually been experienced by the subject. Cook and Campbell refer to this as "assessing whether the treatment manipulation is related to direct measures of the process designed to be affected by the treatment" (p. 60).

Clearly, if the independent variable has not been effectively administered, it cannot be the cause of any change in the dependent variable.

The second area of concern in checking for construct validity involves
what is known as convergent and divergent validity. *Convergent validity* refers to the extent to which the construct is correlated with similar constructs—that is, the extent to which it represents what it is intended to
represent. *Divergent validity* is essentially the reverse—a check to be certain
that your construct is dissimilar from constructs you believe to be unrelated. For example, a researcher would want a new measure of anxiety to
be related to standardized measures of fear and unrelated to measures of
joy or happiness.

A third concern is that the measures used for the dependent variables
("putative effects") tap appropriate factors and that the measures are internally consistent. The level of consistency is determined through comparison of items used to measure the effect and the calculation of a
measure of covariation known as the correlation coefficient (Chapter 13).
Finally, construct validity is facilitated if both the independent and dependent measures are defined narrowly enough to exclude irrelevant factors from the measurement. If such imprecision does exist in the study, it
could obscure the effects of interest. A term frequently applied to such irrelevant, distracting information is "noise." Think of tuning your radio to
your favorite station only to have the signal obscured by static. Even
though the music is there, it is overwhelmed by the noise. In much the
same way, irrelevant factors can serve to mask an effect.

The final type of experimental validity is External Validity. When conducting a study an experimenter hopes to be able to apply the results beyond the immediate situation. This capacity for wide application is known
as generalizability. There are a number of factors that influence whether
such application of results is in fact appropriate. One concern is the sample on which the study was conducted.

When we generalize the results of a study on the effectiveness of transcutaneous electrical stimulation, we want to apply those results to all
those with the characteristics in question, not just to the few we have actually observed. We refer to the entire collection of people sharing a set of
defined characteristics as *the population*. A population is all of any group
we care to define—all patients with Down's syndrome, or all three-year-
old blond girls with autism. Our definition determines the size of the
population.

Generally, our definitions of a population are broad enough that we
can never observe all of the group. We must draw a smaller group—a
sample—and hope our observations of this subset apply to the population.
Since almost all research is conducted on samples, the problem of generalizability or external validity becomes one of some importance. One of

the important controls on external validity involves sampling procedures, as will be discussed later in the chapter.

□ THREATS TO VALIDITY □

Cook and Campbell have identified sources of threats to each of the types of validity discussed above. We will continue our discussion of validity by listing these threats and identifying their sources. Specific research designs have been developed to reduce these threats to validity, and these are discussed in Chapters 4 to 6.

Statistical Conclusion Threats

The seven threats to statistical conclusion validity are: (1) inadequacies in the power of the statistical tests used; (2) violation of the assumptions underlying the tests; (3) 'fishing' and the error rate problem; (4) use of unreliable measures; (5) unreliable implementation of treatment; (6) random irrelevancies in the experimental setting; and (7) random heterogeneity of respondents.

The first three threats involve the choice and implementation of statistical techniques. The first is the *use of statistical tests that lack sufficient power to detect an effect.* Statistical tests vary in their power—that is, in their ability to detect effects. The weaker the effect, the more powerful the technique necessary to observe its presence. Think of trying to see a dim star with your unaided vision, with binoculars, or with a high-powered telescope. The more powerful the instrument, the more likely it is that you will be able to see the star.

In general, statistical techniques of a type known as parametric tests are more powerful than their counterparts, the nonparametric tests. However, parametric tests can be employed only if certain underlying assumptions about the data are satisfied. One of these is that the samples you want to compare have similar variability (homogeneity of variance). If this assumption is not satisfied you must use the less powerful nonparametric tests and risk not detecting an effect that does exist. Failure to do so constitutes the threat of *violation of assumptions of the test statistics.*

Realize, however, that no one is going to physically prevent you from calculating a statistic just because it is not appropriate for the data. Many statistical tests are fairly robust—which means you can stretch the rules about the underlying assumptions without seriously compromising your ability to make appropriate inferences from your results. However, all tests do have limits to their elasticity, and serious violation of assumptions results in seriously incorrect inferences.

As we will discuss in Chapter 11, the game of statistics is in reality a sort of game of chance. We base our statistical conclusions on probabilities of events. So we never know for sure if our inferences are correct. In order to maximize the chances of our being correct, for each test we adopt a criterion of chance—a level of acceptable risk. Usually the level we adopt is .05, which means that 95% of the time we will be correct in drawing conclusions as we have. This level (referred to as the alpha level) holds true for each separate time we calculate a statistic.

Fishing, the third threat to statistical conclusion validity, refers to the unfortunate practice of running every conceivable statistical procedure on a data set in hopes of finding some—any!—effect. (This practice can be traced to the methods used in many academic institutions for determining which members of the faculty will be granted tenure. A primary criterion is often the number of professional publications the faculty member has produced. Hence the phrase, "Publish or perish." Most professional journals will not publish negative results, thus the frantic search for some statistically significant effect.)

Remember, however, that the alpha level (chance of error in our conclusions) refers only to the chance of error for each time a test statistic is calculated. If a researcher fishes through the data and conducts many tests, the chances of one of them coming out significant skyrockets. For example, if three individual tests were performed at .05 alpha level, the three tests as a group would be at an alpha level of .14. An alpha rate of .05 indicates that one time out of 20 the test will appear to be significant even when there is no effect—in other words it will sound a false alarm. Such incorrect conclusions about a study threaten statistical validity.

Reliability of measures and *reliability of treatment implementation* both refer to the concept of experimental reliability to be discussed later in this chapter. Briefly, *reliability* refers to the dependability of a phenomenon. We want to generalize our results only if we believe that the phenomenon we have studied is likely to occur again.

The sixth and seventh sources of threats to statistical validity, *random irrelevancies in the experimental setting* and *random heterogeneity of respondents,* represent two examples of "noise" as defined above—irrelevant factors that detract from or nullify our ability to detect effects. One possible source of such distractions is the setting in which the data are collected. We want to control the environment so as to reduce its effects on our subjects (unless, of course, the environment is our independent variable). We keep the environment as unobtrusive as possible and standardize the environment so that all subjects are exposed to as similar a situation as possible. In this way at least all subjects will be subject to the same influences.

The subjects themselves as human beings possess all sorts of characteristics irrelevant to our research interest. To the extent that factors such as age or gender or diagnosis may affect our dependent measure in some way, these characteristics may also be considered "noise." We can, of course, drastically limit our choice of subjects to reduce interfering influences. When we do this, however, at the same time we increase statistical validity we reduce our external validity. If we want our treatment to be applicable and effective across a broad spectrum of people, we cannot limit the characteristics of our sample.

Threats to Internal Validity

Cook and Campbell list 15 areas in which threats to internal validity can arise: (1) history; (2) maturation; (3) testing; (4) instrumentation; (5) statistical regression; (6) selection; (7) mortality; interactions of selection with (8) maturation, (9) history, and (10) instrumentation; (11) ambiguity about the direction of causal influence; (12) diffusion or imitation of treatments; (13) compensatory equalization of treatments; (14) compensatory rivalry by respondents receiving less desirable treatments; and (15) resentful demoralization of respondents receiving less desirable treatments. In all of these areas, situations can arise in which covariation between variables can be potentially (and plausibly) explained using some phenomenon other than a causal relationship between the variables. These are situations, in other words, that can serve to explain the dependent variable effect without invoking the independent variable cause.

History is a plausible explanation for experimental effects when some outside event that affects outcome measures occurs during the course of a study. Usually this occurrence is conceptualized as a global event that affects more than one or two isolated subjects. In any study that may involve an evaluation, treatment, and further evaluation, some subjects will undergo events that may affect the final evaluation. These events are considered examples of random noise and are expected to even out across subjects. A historical threat to validity might be, say, the replacement of experienced clinicians who perform a pretreatment evaluation of patients' expectations for recovery with inexperienced personnel for post-treatment evaluation. Any change in expectations could be a result of the personnel change.

In some cases the event may be even more global in scope. Americans' attitudes toward gun control underwent a dramatic shift in late 1963 upon the assassination of John F. Kennedy. In the health sciences, news of a breakthrough in treatment of a particular condition might have a similar effect.

Maturation of subjects as a threat to internal validity concerns not events, but the mere passage of time, and therefore may be of particularly serious concern in health science research. As children grow older certain skills appear and develop independent of treatment or training. Patients recovering from an injury may improve and regain strength and mobility independent of treatment as the time since injury increases. The longer

the interval over which treatment occurs, the more plausible is this alternative explanation for observed results.

Testing represents a threat to internal validity in two ways. If the same
instrument is employed in pre-treatment and post-treatment evaluations,
subjects are more familiar with the instrument in the post-treatment situation and usually score higher (although the opposite may also be
found). Familiarity may affect measures such as latency to response or
speed of solution if the test instrument involves any solution algorithm
that the patient may have derived on the first encounter with the instrument. Sheer physical practice may also improve post-treatment scores.

The *instrumentation* employed to measure dependent variables can
threaten internal validity in two ways. First, if the instrument of measurement is a human observer, the instrument itself may exhibit practice effects. As they gain experience, raters tend to perceive phenomena
differently. This may be guarded against by the use of highly trained, experienced observers.

Mechanistic instrumentation such as measurement scales and even
physical equipment may represent instrumentation threats to validity
either if the device is differentially sensitive at various levels along the
range of measurement or if the equipment itself requires (and does not receive) appropriate adjustment and recalibration.

Statistical regression represents an artifact of the testing situation. From
your own experience as a student or as an athlete, you may recall times
when you performed much better than you expected to—when everything went your way—and times when everything that possibly could go
wrong did. Your performance probably evened out over time. Whenever
you evaluate a group of people you will catch some at peaks and some
who probably should not have left the house that day. If you test these
people again—regardless of what you do to them in the interim—things
will also have leveled off for them. Scores will move in the direction of the
"average" score. Thus high initial scores will tend to drop, low initial
scores will tend to increase, and moderate scores will tend to change very
little.

Selection concerns the way in which subjects are placed into experimental groups. Post-treatment comparisons between groups that were not
equivalent initially mean very little. Appropriate sampling procedures (to
be discussed later in this chapter) help to ensure against this threat to
validity.

Mortality of subjects deals with the loss of subjects to the research over
time for various reasons. It is particularly important for the researcher to
note, whenever possible, reasons for the defection of subjects and to pay
especially close attention to attrition rates across experimental conditions.

Selection can combine with other threats to validity to produce selection-maturation, selection-history, and selection-instrumentation inter-

actions. In *selection-maturation* threats the various experimental groups experience maturational change at different rates. A comparison of the improvement in fine motor control over the course of treatment of two-year-old children and eight-year-old children would be confounded by the fact that two-year-olds can be expected to be developing more rapidly than the older children. *Selection-history* is particularly a threat when experimental groups are separated geographically in different states or even different hospitals. An event of local importance may well affect only one of your groups. *Selection-instrumentation* interaction threats occur when experimental groups' average scores differ on an instrument where the intervals are not equal across the entire range of the measure. An example would be a thermometer that was more sensitive below 100 degrees than above 200 degrees.

Ambiguity about the direction of the causal influence is a particularly severe threat in correlational studies where two variables are measured (and not manipulated) and the degree of covariance is calculated. Despite statisticians' repeated warnings about not inferring the direction of causation (or even the existence of causation) from such studies, such inferences are commonly drawn. In some cases logic supplies the intuitively satisfying direction for the relationship. Thus we infer that cigarette smoking causes cancer, not that cancer causes cigarette smoking (although on the basis of the statistical evidence this is an equally correct inference). (Although it is probably true that smoking causes cancer, this conclusion is based on controlled laboratory manipulation, not on correlative statistical relationships between variables.) The temporal sequence of events can also lead researchers to draw incorrect inferences. For this reason, designs that allow the researcher to manipulate the independent variable across initially equivalent experimental groups and then demonstrate differences on the dependent variable are less susceptible to this type of threat.

When the treatment variables consist of some sort of information or training that is intended to be available to only one treatment group, *diffusion of treatment* represents a threat to validity to the extent that individuals from the separate groups have access to and can communicate about the study with each other. As this communication invalidates the intended group differences there remains no cause for any expected effect.

The final three threats to internal validity all involve compensatory activity on the part of either experimenter or subjects that again serves to eliminate intended independent-variable differences between the groups. In *compensatory equalization of treatments*, the researcher—apparently feeling guilty about offering one group a more desirable or effective treatment—lavishes resources on the underprivileged groups, which in effect removes differences in the level of the independent variable. *Compensatory rivalry* by respondents receiving less desirable treatments and *resentful demoralization of respondents* receiving less desirable treatments are two faces of the same coin. In each case the subjects are aware that others are receiving a more effective or desirable treatment. The difference lies in the subjects' response. In the first case this knowledge spurs the subjects into competition with the more privileged subjects. This motivation may create smaller differences between groups than the treatments would appear to indicate. In the second case the underprivileged subjects resentfully resign themselves, and their level of decreased expectation and motivation may result in artificially large differences between the groups.

As can be seen from the above discussion, threats to internal validity may distort the relationship between the experimental variables either by exaggerating or artificially minimizing differences. The unifying theme is that all result in an incorrect belief about the cause and/or effects of the experimental treatments.

Threats to Construct Validity

Threats to construct validity generally involve problems with the theoretical conceptualization of either the independent or dependent variable constructs. The conceptualization may be fuzzy, the construct may be underdeveloped—thereby failing to include important concepts—or the conceptualization may be overambitious to the point of including irrelevant concepts that obscure the core construct. Cook and Campbell list ten threats to construct validity: (1) inadequate preoperational explication of constructs; (2) mono-operational bias; (3) mono-method bias; (4) hypothesis guessing within experimental conditions; (5) evaluation apprehension; 6) experimenter expectancies; (7) confounding constructs and levels of constructs; (8) interaction of different treatments; (9) interaction of testing and treatment; and (10) restricted generalizability across constructs.

Inadequate preoperational explication of constructs consists of the sloppy concepualization referred to above. In this case the researcher does not think through the construct with the thoroughness necessary to clarify the various components of the construct. Experimental variables based on such incomplete preparation manipulate or measure only some aspects of the construct, leaving other aspects untouched. Thus any conclusions drawn from such a study do not fully explore the construct.

Both *mono-operational bias* and *mono-method bias* again involve the variables employed in the research. Every method of manipulating or measuring variables contains an inherent level of error or bias. In order to truly measure a construct the use of multiple methods and operations is highly desirable because the biases of the various methods will tend to cancel each other out, leaving a clearer picture of the construct.

Hypothesis guessing within experimental conditions, evaluation apprehension, and *experimenter expectancies* all involve bias introduced into the measure of the dependent variable. Psychological research has found that subjects are exquisitely sensitive to cues about the researcher's expectations for the outcome of a study and are generally most agreeable in trying to provide just such results. Since the intent of the research is to explore the construct, such cooperation on the part of the subjects is not desirable. On the other hand, some subjects are so apprehensive about being evaluated that their performance suffers to the extent that measures of the dependent variable can be seriously distorted. These threats, which may represent serious problems in research design, are discussed more fully in Chapter 9.

Confounding constructs and levels of constructs is a problem that may occur when the experimenter has failed to recognize that an independent variable construct has several levels that may affect various dependent measures differently. If the experimenter utilizes too few levels of the construct, he or she may incorrectly conclude that the construct itself is not useful.

Some research designs involve exposing subjects to several treatments or manipulations of the independent variable. This is a kind of occurrence that is much more likely in controlled research conditions than in the real world. The threat to construct validity lies in the possibility that the *multiple treatments may interact* in what are known as carry-over effects and provide an effect that is in reality an artifact of the research process rather than an effect of any one treatment.

The *interaction of testing and treatment* again involves a potential contamination of dependent measure responses that is based on experimental procedures. The question in this case is whether the act of testing or evaluating in itself affects the response to the treatment variables. If so, then the measures of the dependent variable do not reflect the effect of the independent variable, but rather the effect of the way the testing has been done.

The final threat to construct validity, *restricted generalizability across constructs*, involves imprecise conceptualization of constructs in that the study designer has not given adequate thought to the question of which dependent measure the independent variable construct could be expected to influence. If the researcher has not considered this problem, the study may collect inappropriate dependent measures and incorrect conclusions may be drawn about the construct operationalized by the independent variable.

Construct validity is essential to good research. If the basic issues of the study have not been thoroughly considered and constructs appropriately defined and measured, the researcher cannot hope to draw scientifically sound conclusions.

Threats to External Validity

External validity refers to the extent to which experimental findings can be applied to situations outside the research setting. Cook and Campbell identify three threats to generalizability, all of which involve the interaction of the treatment with another factor. The threats are (1) interaction of selection and treatment; (2) interaction of setting and treatment; and (3) interaction of history and treatment.

Particularly in research involving clinical treatment methods, an important concern is whether patients outside the research setting will respond in the same way as research subjects. It is important, then, to ensure that research subjects are representative of the population. Methods to increase the typicalness of subjects are discussed later in this chapter in the section on sampling techniques. Use of these methods reduces the probability of the threat posed by the *interaction of selection and treatment*. A particular threat to external validity is the use of volunteer subjects. Volunteers often have characteristics that differ from those of the general population. For example, in the pioneering studies by Masters and Johnson on human sexuality, subjects provided information on their sexual behavior and performed sexual acts in the laboratory. A wealth of new knowledge was provided on the physiology of human sexual response. Yet in terms of attitudes and behaviors, how typical of the general population were these subjects?

The threat of the *interaction of setting and treatment* involves the extent to which the experimental setting resembles the setting in which treatment will be received in post-experimental situations. This problem is less severe in the health sciences than in, say,the behavioral and social sciences, where college students often serve as subjects for research intended to be generalized to industrial or other non-academic settings. The control and similarity of medical care facilities minimizes this threat for health science professionals.

The *interaction of history and treatment* involves differences in the ways that various treatment groups may be affected by events occurring during the course of the research. For example, the treatment might be either enhanced or sabotaged by an outside event while the control group remains unaffected.

At this point you may be wondering how researchers ever manage to design a completely valid study. The truth is that no one ever does. There is no perfect study, only studies containing degrees of imperfection. This is why studies must be replicated in other settings, by other researchers, using other operations and methods. Good researchers are constantly aware of the pitfalls of study design presented by threats to validity and try to avoid as many of them as possible.

□ RELIABILITY □

In the experimental context, the concept of reliability involves several related issues. In all cases the common-usage notion of reliability as trustworthiness is applicable. A person or phenomenon is reliable when we can count on the stability of certain occurrences or characteristics. Science is in a very real way based on the concept of reliability. Prediction is possible only because of the dependability of events. In a world where events were random and unstable we could never with any certainty anticipate phenomena—even the rising of the sun. In a basically reliable world, then, scientists seek to ensure (1) the reliability of experimental measures; (2) the reliability of the implementation of treatments in research settings; and—probably the most important—(3) the reliability of results.

The issue of the reliability of experimental measures assumes that the phenomenon or characteristic to be measured is itself stable and reliable. Take, for example, the situation in which a thermometer is employed to determine a patient's temperature. Three different readings over a three-hour period yield the following results: 98.6, 95, and 109. You would probably conclude the thermometer in question was inaccurate and unreliable. Why? Because we know that a human being's body temperature is not that variable. We draw the conclusion that the problem lies with the instrument of measurement.

It was easy to assess the reliability of the thermometer in the example above because of our knowledge of the phenomenon being measured. Very often in research we do not have such a clear picture of the experimental constructs. Thus reliability is to some extent related to construct validity. A thoroughly conceptualized, well-defined construct employed as the independent variable enhances our ability to determine the reliability of measures designed to quantify the dependent measure.

Whenever we utilize a measurement device, the data we obtain—the patients' body temperature or grip strength or expectations for recovery—consist of two components. One component is the actual information we seek, the other is what is known as error of measurement. No measuring instrument measures exactly and exclusively the phenomenon of interest. Perhaps the instrument is not sufficiently sensitive to the phenomenon, or the range is too broad, or the very act of inquiring about an attitude changes (or creates) the attitude. In creating measurement devices, we seek to minimize the error of measurement so we can focus our attention on the phenomenon of interest.

Researchers employ a number of techniques to test the reliability of variable measures. All involve a statistical technique known as correlation. As you will recall from our discussion of the ambiguity about the direction of causal influence, correlation measures the extent of covariation between measures. (For a more complete discussion, see Chapter 13). In the testing of reliability, the measures consist of a pair of scores on a pair of measures of interest.

Instrument Reliability

There are basically three types of instrument reliability of interest to researchers. The first type is concerned with reliability of scores across a time interval and includes test-retest and alternate form reliability. The second type of reliability is concerned with the purity of the measure and with internal consistency in measures such as questionnaires. Methods include split-half reliability. Finally, when observers or raters are used in a study, there is the question of inter-rater reliability—that is, the extent to which individuals perceive a person or phenomenon similarly.

Test-retest reliability is precisely what the name implies. Subjects are measured on some characteristic, an interval of time is allowed to elapse, then subjects are re-evaluated with the same measurement instrument. The scores of the two administrations are then tested for covariation using the statistical technique known as correlation. Assuming that the phenomenon being studied is stable, scores should not vary much. We will still find some regression toward the mean among extreme initial scores and a certain unavoidable amount of random fluctuation as a result of such irrelevant human frailties as being tired or bored or ill. We would expect these noise factors to balance out across subjects.

A variation on the measurement of reliability over time is the use of alternate forms of measure at the measurement points. Subjects' scores on the parallel instruments are then correlated. Although finding equivalent yet different measures may be difficult, this approach has several advantages. First, you need not worry whether familiarity with the test or practice is affecting re-test scores. Also, by operationalizing your measures differently you are increasing the chances of construct validity by avoiding a duplication of measurement biases and errors.

Split-half reliability concerns the extent to which components of a measure are evaluating the same phenomenon. Here again we are faced with a question of construct validity. In a questionnaire or interest inventory, if diverse, unrelated concepts are being tapped, the instrument may not actually measure the construct of interest. It may measure something wholly irrelevant. Hence we want an internally consistent, well conceptualized measure. To assess this type of reliability, researchers divide the questions or items from one administration of the test into two groups and compare a subject's score on the two halves of the test to gain a measure of split-half reliability. Usually the division is accomplished by placing even-numbered items into one group and odd-numbered items into the other. This technique helps to even out any irrelevant environmental or personal noise, such as time of day, temperature of room, or tiredness, which might appear if the first half of the test were compared with the second half. If the scores of the two halves of the test are similiar, the instrument is considered reliable.

The assessment of inter-rater reliability is intended to ensure that individual observers rate the same phenomenon in the same way. There are basically two types of inter-rater reliability. The first involves a rater's consistency with him or herself. Recall that reliability refers to stability. A rater exposed to a phenomenon on two separate occasions should show consistency in rating just as we expect reliability from an inanimate instrument such as a thermometer. One way to increase a rater's inter-rating reliability is to ensure that any raters employed in a study have reached a defined standard of experience and expertise before they are used in the study. This will help protect against errors that might arise as a result of changes in proficiency.

When using several raters in a study (from a design standpoint a very sound approach, since it minimizes the idiosyncrasies potentially inherent in any one individual's ratings) we have to be concerned not only with each rater's consistency with her or himself, but also with consistency with other raters. Instruments should rate the same phenomenon similarly. Large inter-rater differences in ratings introduce larger than acceptable amounts of measurement error. Inter-rater reliability should be assessed at several points in the study just as you would recheck several times the calibration of a mechanical instrument.

Standardization of the Treatment of Subjects

The second major area of interest to research designers ensuring the reliability of a study is concerned with the standardization of treatment of subjects. If we wish to assess the effects of manipulating the independent variable, we must be certain that subjects in each group received the treatment as specified. The concern is biased treatment of groups, which can result in dependent-variable differences between the groups that are not relevant to the study. Have we controlled for outside influences? Are all members of an experimental group being treated identically? Such factors as standardization of instructions, time of day of measurement, person conducting the measurement, temperature of the room can all introduce irrelevant influences. Just as all members within a group should receive standard treatment, the only difference between the research groups should be the level of the independent variable. If we find differences on the dependent measures between initially equivalent groups whose only difference is the level of independent variable, we have a strong case for the effectiveness of our treatment as opposed to alternative explanations.

Perhaps the most important guarantee of study reliability is the assurance that the levels of treatment were implemented as specified by the research proposal. It is most difficult to assess or argue the effectiveness of a treatment that has not been administered. A great deal of thought and creativity on the part of the researcher goes into standardizing and controlling all other aspects of the study in order to highlight treatment differences, so it is essential these differences do in fact exist.

Stability of Obtained Results

The final—and most serious—aspect of experimental reliability refers to the stability or trustworthiness of the obtained results. In part this is a statistical issue, in that we base our decision as to whether an effect is "significant" (or reliable) on the laws of probability, not on some omniscient access to reality. What we really want to know is, "If I were to conduct this same study again would I obtain the same results?" If the answer is "no" we may have wasted our time (as well as other resources). If the answer is "yes" we can generalize our results across time and across appropriately controlled environments. This ability to make inferences about a population on the basis of sample data is the cornerstone of external validity and, indeed, of the entire scientific research process.

The concepts of reliability and validity are inextricably interrelated. If we do not have construct validity, it is irrelevant whether our instruments are reliable. However, even if our constructs are valid, we must employ reliable measures if we wish to draw any conclusions about the effects of our treatments. The threat to internal validity presented by instrumentation involves the reliability of measuring instruments. As discussed above, effects based on changes in the measures themselves destroy the validity of inferences about treatment effectiveness. Statistical validity and external validity both relate to the concept of the reliability of statistical conclusions. If we wish to generalize our results we must have employed appropriate statistical techniques and decision-making procedures. Only then can we assume not only that our results are not illusory but also that they would apply in other settings.

□ SAMPLING □

The issue of choosing a research sample has arisen during the discussion of three of our types of validity. Appropriate sampling techniques reduce the threats posed by (1) random heterogeneity of respondents (which threatens statistical validity); (2) selection interactions, such as selection–maturation, selection–history, selection–instrumentation (which threaten internal validity); and (3) interactions between selection and treatment (which threaten external validity). The sampling process involves two steps: choosing the subjects to serve in our study, and determining which subjects receive which treatment.

When choosing subjects to participate in our research, we have two types of sampling techniques from which to choose. In probability sampling, decisions are based on random selection. This means that each element in the population has an equal, independent probability of becoming a subject in the study. This random assignment seeks to randomize irrelevant factors (noise) across experimental conditions and to create a group of subjects very similar to the population in order to increase external validity.

Probability Sampling

There are four major types of probability sampling: (1) simple random sampling, (2) stratified random sampling, (3) systematic sampling, and (4) cluster sampling.

Simple random sampling is the purest form of sampling from a theoretical standpoint but is often unworkable because of practical factors. In simple random sampling the first step is to define the population of interest. Clearly, limiting the definition of the population will make it easier to acquire a representative random sample of subjects, yet limiting the definition of the population may severely limit the external validity of the study. For example, you could define your population as children with cerebral palsy or children under the age of five years with cerebral palsy who are patients at Anytown General Hospital. You clearly have more access in the second case, but you should have concerns about whether this narrow group is typical of the larger population.

Once the population is defined, and a complete list of the elements in the population is compiled, subjects are chosen for inclusion in the study through a random choice process. If the group is small enough, lots can be drawn. For larger populations, a table of random numbers may be employed. Randomization will be discussed in Chapter 4. The primary concern in this method is that the listing of the population being used in the choice process be complete. An example of a situation where listing presents a problem is the use of the telephone directory as the listing of the population for an attitude survey—*unless* the population is defined as people with telephones who are willing to allow their numbers to be publicly listed. Using phone book listings to represent the general population is an error because, as a group, people listed in the phone book probably possess characteristics that render them atypical (in this case, the possession of at least enough money to have a telephone independent of factors that would result in an unlisted number). No matter how correct your sampling procedures, your sample will not be appropriately random when chosen from an improperly listed population.

Stratified random sampling techniques are appropriate when your population is divided into subgroups that should be represented in your sample. For example, if you could somehow list the entire population of the world and randomly selected two groups of people, in theory you would have an equal number of men and women in your groups. However, it is theoretically possible that all of one group could be male and all of the other female (even though the odds against it are astronomical). If you had reason to believe that gender affected the response to treatment, you would not want to utilize such nonequivalent groups.

In this case you would stratify your population into separate listings of men and women and make your random choices from these lists. If the strata or subgroups make up unequal proportions of the population, you would match these proportions in your sample, using a technique known as proportional stratified sampling. This method maximizes external validity by assuring a sample representative of the population.

There is no sampling error on the stratified variable—that is, there is perfect representation on the stratified variable. This, in turn, enhances the representativeness of the other variables related to the stratified variable. Therefore, a stratified random sample is likely to be more representative than a simple random sample.

In systematic sampling, the researcher chooses subjects from the population through the use of a model or system. Every *k*th element in the population is chosen for inclusion. The researcher must very carefully define the population. Should you include every third aphasic patient or every fifth ambulatory patient? Again you must balance convenience, construct definition, and external validity issues.

Cluster sampling involves the successive random sampling from units of successively decreasing size. For example, if we wanted to sample from all physical therapists in the United States employed in health care facilities, we would start by randomly sampling from the 50 states. Once we had chosen our subgroup of states, we would choose another subgroup from the counties in those states. In our chosen counties we would randomly sample hospitals and health care facilities and obtain a listing of physical therapists in those facilities. Cluster sampling represents a variation on simple random sampling in that each physical therapist employed in a health care facility began our hypothetical sampling procedure with an equal probability of inclusion into the sample. Cluster sampling is efficient, but you pay for this efficiency in terms of accuracy. A single, random sample from a population is subject to a single sample error. Each stage of cluster sampling allows for additional sampling error.

Nonprobability Sampling Techniques

Although probability sampling procedures are theoretically far superior, there is also another group of sampling procedures, known as nonprobability techniques. These techniques are generally inferior in that they often introduce sources of bias into the sample. Generalizability of results based on nonprobability sampling is often very questionable. In general, anything the researcher can do to employ probability techniques will improve the quality of the research, even if to do so requires narrowing the population definition.

The first type of nonprobability sampling is known as quota sampling. Quota sampling is much like stratified random sampling in that the population is stratified into subgroups before selection of subjects. The choice of subjects from the strata, however, is not random. The researcher instead employs some subjective (and potentially biasing) selection procedure.

In purposive sampling the researcher depends entirely on his or her judgment (and subjectivity) to select subjects. The researcher purposely examines and selects subjects whom he or she feels are typical or representative of a particular constellation of characteristics. This method of selection is tremendously sensitive to the biases and judgment of the researcher. The researcher hopes (often incorrectly) that errors in judgment in the selection will tend to counterbalance each other.

In terms of providing a typical or generalizable sample, probably the worst type of nonprobability sampling is the use of the sample of convenience. In this method the researcher makes use of a group of subjects readily at hand regardless of their characteristics or similarity to the population. The use of volunteers is an example of this type of sampling. Please don't misunderstand: All subjects must eventually agree to participate in research or their use is unethical. A volunteer is someone who comes forward and asks to be involved in the research without any prior selection on the part of the researcher. Volunteers represent a very suspect source of data. Why did this particular group of people want to be in the study? How do they differ from nonvolunteers? The answers to these questions may well call into question the external validity of a study.

A variation on the use of the sample of convenience is known as snowball sampling. The first group of subjects in the study (who themselves are probably volunteers) are asked if they know anyone who might wish to participate in the study. In this way subjects recruit other subjects. This can be particularly biasing to the results of the study if subjects disclose too much about the study. (Recall that diffusion of treatments was discussed as a threat to internal validity.) In addition, the researcher has very little control over the types of person who may be recruited by previous subjects.

Sample Size

One question that we have ignored up to now is the number of subjects we should select. A glib and not terribly useful reply would be "enough." The major factors controlling how many subjects are enough are based on statistical and practical concerns.

We must be concerned with sample size for several reasons. We perform statistical techniques on samples we believe to be similar to the population. Thus when we calculate statistics for our sample we assume the values obtained are close to the values we could calculate if we had access to the entire population. Sample size directly affects the amount of confidence we can have in that assumption. The error in approximation is generally larger for small samples. The larger the sample (as a proportion of the population) the more accurate the approximation.

Several of the most powerful and most commonly used statistical procedures rest on certain assumptions about the distribution of the data set (these tests are known as parametric tests and are discussed in Chapters 12 and 13). If these assumptions are not met, the results of the technique are useless. One of the assumptions is that the shape of the data population is "normal." We're using this term in a very precise manner. A normal curve (also known as a bell-shaped curve) is a symmetrical distribution possessing very useful mathematical qualities. Many phenomena naturally possess a normal distribution. When we sample repeatedly from almost any distribution, however, whether normal or skewed, if our sample is large enough, the graph of the distribution of the sample means will have a normal shape, and parametric techniques may be appropriately employed. There are some limitations on when it is appropriate to assume this property for sample distributions, and these are delineated in a theorem known as the Central Limit Theorem. One consequence of this theorem is that you must have at least 30 subjects in each of your smallest subgroupings if you are going to use parametric tests.

You will notice in the previous sentence that the size of the smallest subgroup of interest is the number you should take most seriously. This is an argument for keeping studies relatively simple, because the requisite number of subjects increases at an appalling rate with the inclusion of each new factor. If, for example, you are comparing the effectiveness of comprehensive stroke rehabilitation and general medical rehabilitation in the treatment of stroke and you think that age and onset may influence effectiveness, your smallest subgroup would be recent onset patients receiving comprehensive stroke rehabilitation treatment. If you are going to use parametric tests, you will need at least 30 such patients.

Up to this point it may appear as if increasing the number of subjects is always a desirable course to pursue. There exists at least one situation in which too large a number of subjects may actually be undesirable.

For most statistical tests the determination of whether or not our treatment was effective is based on the statistical significance of the results (that is, on the likelihood of the observed effects being the result of chance alone). In many tests, the greater the number of subjects used, the smaller is the effect (or group difference) necessary to declare the results significant. For one statistical technique, however, statistical and practical significance may well be essentially unrelated. A correlation (Chapter 13) measures the extent of covariation between two measures. By squaring the value of the correlation coefficient, r, we obtain a measure called the coefficient of determination, or r^2. If I obtain an r^2 of .80 between two measures I know that 80% of the variability in one measure is related to variability in the other measure. If I have enough subjects, an r of .10 may be statistically significant. However, since the coefficient of determination, r^2, is .01, I am not accounting for 99% of the variability in my measures. So paying too much attention or attaching too much importance to statistical significance in this case would be unwise. In this case indiscriminately increasing the sample size would not be appropriate.

Let's stop being statistically prissy and be practical for a moment. Suppose you don't have access to unlimited numbers of subjects appropriate for your research? This is a very salient question because that will often be the case. What then? All is not lost. Nonparametric tests are not as powerful as parametric tests, but they will do the job when necessary. You can also increase the strength of the treatment (manipulation of the independent variable) to increase the size of the effect.

In practical terms the researcher may be constrained by limits associated with the availability and cost of subjects. If you are studying a rare phenomenon you will be limited in terms of numbers. If the experimental procedures per subject are expensive in terms of money or time required you will be limited by cost. These are both realistic limitations on sample size.

A final influence on sample size involves experimental mortality. How many subjects can be expected to complete the study? If the procedures take place over a long period, as in a longitudinal study, the experimenter must build in an excess of subjects initially to ensure enough data at the end of the study. Mail-in questionnaire studies are often plagued with a return rate as low as 35% to 40%. Assuming some of the returned forms are unusable because subjects did not follow directions, a researcher must distribute approximately 150 forms in order to be sure of getting 50 usable responses. This return rate problem is difficult to solve. Providing incentives such as remuneration for compliance may increase the return rate, but may also alter the motivation of subjects and possibly interfere with the validity of the study's results.

Assignment of Subjects

Once we have decided on our sample size and chosen our subjects we must (in many types of designs) assign them to different treatment groups or conditions. Researchers have basically three alternative methods of assignment to condition.

Simple random assignment is precisely what the name implies. Subjects are chosen from the group of subjects in the study and randomly assigned to condition. This means that each subject is equally likely to be assigned to each of the study's groups. If the study subjects represent subgroups, stratified sampling procedures may be employed.

The second method of assignment is known as matched random assignment. After the initial subject group is selected, pairs of subjects are matched on characteristics that might affect the dependent measure but are irrelevant to the independent measure. For example, subjects in a study on the effectiveness of weight-loss programs might be expected to lose amounts of weight dependent on their initial weight. A subject with 100 pounds to lose might be expected to lose more weight than one with

10 pounds to lose. The experimenter would match pairs based on initial weight so that each subject with 10 or 50 or 100 pounds to lose had a counterpart in the other group(s). This method ensures the equivalence of the treatment groups.

The use of matched pairs across groups helps to control irrelevant factors. The ultimate in this form of control is the repeated-measures design. Here a subject is exposed to all experimental conditions, and scores across conditions are compared. Since a subject's characteristics such as gender, age, and temperament remain constant across all conditions, they are removed as plausible explanations for differences on the dependent variable. This technique is also known as using the subject as his or her own control.

If this design is so terrific, you might ask, why is it not employed most, if not all the time? If you consider the weight-loss example cited above, you will see one difficulty. If weight-loss Program A is effective and Jane Doe loses 100 pounds, how likely (or ethical) would it be that we could persuade her to regain the weight to try Program B? Or, if she didn't lose on Program A but subsequently lost on Program B, was the loss the result of B alone, or in combination with Program A? Because of such carry-over effects even when repeated measures are possible, treatments are administered in different orders to different subjects. If one treatment still appears more effective in this counterbalanced design we can feel more confident that we are seeing treatment and not order effects.

The issues of validity, reliability, and sampling are interrelated concerns that underlie all of scientific research. Various specific research designs have been developed to deal with these issues. Chapters 4 through 6 describe these basic designs and Chapters 12 and 13 describe the statistical procedures appropriate for specific designs.

□ SUMMARY □

Validity is the research concept that pertains to the accuracy of the research. Four types of validity must be considered: (1) internal validity, which refers to the relationship between variables in the study; (2) statistical conclusion validity, which refers to the appropriate choices and applications of analytic procedures; (3) construct validity of putative causes and effects, which involves the conceptualization and measurement of theoretical constructs in the research; and (4) external validity, which refers to the generalizability of research results. Threats to validity provide plausible explanations for research findings other than the research hypothesis and are thus to be carefully avoided.

Reliability refers to the stability of research measures. It is important for the statistical reliability of results that the measures employed in data collection and treatment implementation have this stability.

Appropriate sampling procedures enhance both the validity and the reliability of research findings. The unbiased selection of subjects and assignment to condition increases the likelihood that the sample approximates the population of interest, thus increasing the generalizability of results.

□ KEY TERMS □

validity
statistical conclusion validity
internal validity
construct validity
external validity
sample
reliability
test-retest reliability
split half reliability
inter-rater reliability

probability sampling
simple random sampling
systematic sampling
cluster sampling
nonprobability sampling
quota sampling
purposive sampling
convenience sampling
snowball sampling
random assignment

□ 4 □
Pre-Experimental and Experimental Designs

We have finally reached a point in our research odyssey where we must decide on the actual structure of the study we will employ to test our hypotheses. In the next three chapters we will explore the three major groupings of designs: true experimental designs, quasi-experimental designs, and nonexperimental designs. Purely from a research design standpoint, these groupings represent decreasing levels of desirability. In practical terms, however, it is often simply not possible to exercise the control necessary to employ a true experimental design, and one of the other design types must be used, with the loss of a certain amount of control. The costs associated with this loss in control include a seriously compromised ability to identify the source of any experimental effects.

□ CHARACTERISTICS OF TRUE EXPERIMENTS □

Up to this time we have used the words *research* and *experiment* more or less interchangeably. While this blurring of distinctions is common in everyday usage, it is technically incorrect. Experiments are one type of research, but, as mentioned above, only one type. To avoid any possible confusion, the term *experiment* will be qualified as to type when it refers to a specific design. The un-qualified form will continue to refer to the more general research process.

What is it that characterizes true experiments and makes them preferred over other forms of research? True experiments constitute the tightest, most precise form of research and allow us to have the most confidence in our results. True experiments possess three defining characteristics: manipulation, control, and randomization. If a design lacks any of these factors it is pre-experimental (lacking randomization), quasi-experimental (lacking control or randomization), or non-experimental (lacking manipulation).

Manipulation

Manipulation is the basic characteristic that distinguishes the various types of experimental research from non-experimental research. For research to be considered experimental, the researcher must do something to subjects (manipulate the levels of the independent variable) in order to assess effects on the dependent variable. Clearly, it is simpler to manipulate the independent variable when we are dealing with an active independent variable—that is, an independent variable in which the researcher assigns subjects to the group or level variable. The researcher can assign various types of treatment, for example, or amounts of treatment or medication.

Often, however, the researcher is interested in differences in the levels of an independent variable that is an attribute, such as age, gender, or diagnosis. The researcher cannot manipulate such variables but instead must assign individuals to their naturally occurring groups. When a researcher is employing only one independent variable and that independent variable is an attribute, the research is by definition non-experimental.

It is possible (and often desirable) to employ more than one independent variable in a study. In this case an attribute variable might become an intervening variable. In a study on patient compliance (defined as how closely a patient adheres to a schedule of exercises outside the health care setting) the researcher might manipulate the types of instructions given patients in an attempt to ensure (or increase) compliance—in other words, Type of Instruction is the independent variable. Some patients might receive a talk that points out all of the benefits and positive points of compliance, while others may be presented with all of the damage and dangers associated with noncompliance.

The researcher might further believe that patients of different ages will respond to the two instruction sets differently—might believe, in other words, that age will be an intervening variable. The patients might then be divided into three groups, under 30 years of age, 30-60 years of age, and over 60 years of age. The subjects in each group of patients would be randomly divided into two subgroups and randomly assigned to receive either the reward or the threat instructions. Even though age was not manipulated, this study qualifies as a true experiment because of the manipulation of instructions and the random assignment of subjects to groups of equal age distribution.

Control

The second hallmark of the true experiment is control. Control is basically the measure of the experimenter's ability to eliminate irrelevant influences and information from the study in order to eliminate any plausible explanations for results other than the independent variable manipulation. In effect, then, control subsumes manipulation and randomization. The experimenter must eliminate noise both from the construct of the independent variable and from the implementation of the variables. Randomization seeks to increase experimental control through equalizing noise in the experimental groups by ensuring that groups will be equivalent at the beginning of the study.

Since noise in research can be caused by any number of outside influences, the research laboratory represents the epitome of control. In the laboratory the experimenter can exercise control over such potentially intervening variables as room temperature, level of illumination, or color of walls. All of these variables have been seen to influence people's reactions. If, as the experimenter, I can absolutely control the experience of my subjects and I know the only difference between the way the groups were treated was the manipulation of my independent variable, I will be comfortable in claiming that any observed group differences (or changes in an individual pre- to post-treatment) were based on my treatment.

One way in which experimenters increase control is through the use of the control group. If I want to test the effectiveness of a new type of treatment the only way I can assess effectiveness is by using a comparison. Is my treatment better than nothing? Better than alternative treatments? The use of a control group provides a baseline for comparison.

Usually the control group receives no treatment. Thus I would choose two equivalent groups, treat one, then compare the groups on the dependent measure(s). If the control group's scores on my measure are similar to the experimental group's scores, I would probably have to fail to reject the null hypothesis. I could not conclude that my treatment had an effect.

In a medical setting, the use of strictly defined control groups may conflict with medical ethics. Is it ethical to allow patients in need of treatment to go untreated for research purposes? Often the answer to that question is "no." In such a case our control group will assume a different character. Since what is needed is a comparison, a new treatment might be administered to the experimental group while the control group receives whatever the standard treatment had been. Under these conditions, the study addresses a slightly different research question. Instead of assessing whether a treatment works, this design assesses whether the new treatment is more effective. In practice, this second question is probably the more important one.

Randomization

Researchers employ randomization techniques to reduce systematic bias in a study and thus increase its internal validity. Randomization reduces the risk of threats to internal validity stemming from mortality, maturation, testing, regression, and selection bias. When we even out subjects' characteristics across conditions through randomization we should be evening out the factors that result in differences in attrition across groups, in developmental rates, and in responses to testing. In addition, we ensure, as far as possible, that unusually high or low scores, which we could expect to regress toward the mean, will be evenly distributed between the groups, and, by definition, we have reduced selection threats by increasing the probability that our groups are equivalent to begin with. As you may recall from Chapter 3, we randomize selection and assignment of subjects not only to increase the probability that our groups will be equivalent at the beginning of the study but also to increase external validity: The more our research groups are typical of individuals in the population to which we wish to generalize our results, the more safely may we do so.

In some situations, randomization of assignment to treatment provides benefits beyond research design considerations. When the treatment under consideration represents a potential breakthrough in terms of effectiveness, and the supply of the treatment is limited, choosing individuals to receive the better treatment presents an ethical dilemma. The fairest way to distribute services in such situations may well be to use randomization in choosing those who will receive the limited resources.

By this point in the discussion, randomization may have begun to seem like a panacea for research design ills. It is important to point out that although randomization usually helps reduce sources of bias, the randomization process is not perfect. Randomization is most effective in equalizing groups when we have a large number of subjects to assign to each condition, or when we are choosing large samples from the population. The randomization process is based on the laws of probability. Sometimes improbable events occur. It is possible our groups will still include sources of bias even when randomly chosen and assigned. Just by chance we might find all of our older, or more intelligent, or more tolerant patients are assigned to one group.

Above and beyond such potential inherent bias, another source of bias may be inappropriate use of the methods of randomization. To be completely random, each element must have an equal, independent probability of selection or assignment to group. Use of sloppy methods may alter this element of equal probability. An unfortunate example of such a situation occurred in 1969 when the United States moved to the use of a lottery to determine order of conscription of young men into the military. Slips representing dates of birth were placed in an urn and drawn for order. Had the slips been properly mixed, each month should have had an equal probability of being drawn early. Instead, dates in the last three months (December, November, and October) were over-represented in the early drawing, totaling 9 of the first 25 dates drawn. The probability of this event happening by chance is remote (50,000 to 1, according to McClavae & Benson, 1985).

As we proceed to a discussion of methods of randomization, then, bear in mind that randomization presents the best alternative for reducing initial bias in research, but that even with proper procedures properly conducted, some inequities may exist based on the laws of probability. Careful researchers will often take measures on their experimental groups pre- treatment as well as post-treatment to assess statistically whether the groups were initially equivalent.

The Process of Randomization The actual physical implementation of randomization may be accomplished in several ways. As can be seen from the example of the U.S. Selective Service (the draft), when the number of elements is small, the elements may be drawn from a hat or an urn. Even in the case of small numbers, however, bias can enter the system. The slips or elements may be improperly mixed, or a slip may stick to the side of the urn. Generally it is preferable to employ a table of random numbers.

Tables of random numbers are usually generated by computer. They consist of the digits from 0 to 9 arranged in such a way that each digit is equally likely to appear next in the sequence. A portion of a random numbers table appears in Table 4-1.

TABLE 4-1 TABLE OF
RANDOM NUMBERS

1333	0051	0888	7835
3197	→ 4325	2683	7360
0699	5950	0239	8655
8497	9818	2420	9945
9298	5468	8452	7985
2238	4415	0332	3070

When employing a random number table in the selection of subjects for research, the experimenter first needs a complete listing of the population. In cases where the population is quite large, obviously this in itself presents a problem. However, in such cases methods such as random cluster sampling might be employed. For the sake of an example, let's say we're interested in the attitudes of practicing occupational therapists toward the increased emphasis on research in OT education. We would want to choose a sample to which to address our questions. If we believe that most American OTs belong to the American Occupational Therapy Association, we might use their membership listing as the basis for our sample selection. (To some extent this does represent a sample of convenience. Most applied research grapples with this problem of appropriate sampling.)

With our listing in one hand and our table of random numbers in the other, we're ready to begin. First, I would enter the table of random numbers by arbitrarily pointing to some place on the page. I would use this number to determine on which page of the AOTA listing I would begin sampling. Since the digits are random, I can proceed in any direction I choose from my initial starting point for my next digit. Suppose my initial choice was a 4 (as indicated by the arrow in the table) and, (moving to the right) my next digit was a 3. This would tell me I should begin on the fourth page of the listing with the third name on the page. (Digits may be used singly or in combinations with equal correctness.)

Still moving to the right, I decide to use two digit numbers to select the sample names. My next two-digit number is a 25, so I skip to the 25th name after my initial subject. I continue in this manner until I have chosen the desired number of subjects.

Let's imagine that I suspected that expressed attitudes toward research training might depend on the type of methodology employed to gather data from the subjects. To cover this condition, I decide to send one-third of my subjects written questionnaires, to contact one-third by telephone, and to interview one-third in person. Now I must assign my subjects to one of the three conditions. My first step is to divide the sample into the three groups. Only then will I determine, by random assignment, which group receives which treatment.

To achieve this random assignment, we begin with a list of the subjects. Let's say I have chosen 90 names. I assign a number from 1 to 90 to each subject. Then I enter my table of random numbers at some new arbitrary point and proceed until I reach a number falling between 1 and 90. The individual from my list matched with this number becomes my first subject in my first condition. The subject whose number I encounter second becomes the first subject in my second condition and so on, rotating through the three conditions until all subjects are assigned to a group.

The final step is to number by conditions—questionnaires becomes 1, telephone interviews becomes 2, and personal interviews becomes 3. I enter the table one more time to assign the groups to the conditions. I will assign my first sample group to the condition whose number I encounter first. Thus if I first come across a 3, Group 1 receives personal interviews. I continue through the table until I encounter either a 1 or a 2, which then determines the assignments of the remaining conditions. By employing randomization techniques at each step of the process, I have greatly enhanced the probable internal and external validity of my study.

Checks on Randomization   Recall that, by chance, my groups may not be equivalent despite the use of randomization procedures. It is wise for the experimenter to make use of several techniques to assess both initial equivalence and any possible effects of mortality on the equivalence of conditions.

To continue with our example on attitudes toward research training, we would want to take the time to consider what subject characteristics might influence attitudes. Let's say we decide age, length of time since training, and geographical location might bias attitudes. We would then wish to look at our groups to see if these characteristics were evenly distributed. We might not be able to assess all of the factors of interest from our source (in this case the AOTA listing). In that case we would want to build into our research instrument questions on these factors. Once we have the information at our disposal, we can employ a nonparametric statistical test known as the chi square test, which will tell us if our groups are, in fact, equivalent in composition. (Having this information bolsters later inferences, so it is wise to take the time for this step.)

In some studies we could go so far as to pre-test our research groups on our dependent measures before our experimental manipulation. Then we not only have before and after measures to assess change within the groups, we also have the means to compare the groups pre- and post-treatment. In our example, because we are studying the measurement process itself, such methods are not usable.

Careful researchers run checks to ascertain that initially equivalent groups remain equivalent throughout the study. In our example we were planning to start out with 15 subjects in each of our three groups. We could not realistically expect that we could collect useable data on all subjects. We would want to carefully examine the characteristics of those subjects who leave the study. If we found that only the youngest subjects returned questionnaires and only the older subjects agreed to be interviewed, our results might be due to age differences—not method differences. It is wise, therefore, whenever possible to check for equivalence both before the experimental manipulation and after data collection before statistical analysis. (Statistical techniques that can aid in controlling for some group nonequivalence are discussed in Chapter 12.)

□ FIELD VS LABORATORY EXPERIMENTS □

Earlier in our discussion of control we extolled the virtues of the research laboratory. At this point an explicit distinction should be drawn between laboratory and field experiments. As discussed previously, the laboratory excels in the potential for control in experiments. It is essentially an artificial environment created especially for research. But the increase in control is not without cost. The tighter the experimental control, the less the environment resembles the real world. Thus external validity may suffer. The laboratory is much more suited for basic than for applied research.

Field experiments are conducted in the real world. No special environment is constructed. This may greatly lessen experimental control. But, again, the trade-off may be greatly enhanced external validity. Since most applied research deals with a real-world situation, field experiments are often employed for this type of research. The lack of control can become a serious problem: lack of control is one of the characteristics that distinguishes between true and quasi-experimental designs. Poorly controlled experiments must be considered quasi-experiments.

□ EXPERIMENTAL DESIGNS □

We will begin this discussion of experimental designs (based on Campbell & Stanley, 1963) with three examples of poor research design (pre-experimental designs), which will be contrasted with more acceptable designs (true experimental designs). To simplify explanations, we will adopt Campbell and Stanley's system of notation. An X will represent an experimental treatment or manipulation, an O the fact that an observation or measurement takes place, and an R the fact that randomization procedures will be employed. The temporal sequence will move from left to right, so the notation $X\ O$ indicates a treatment followed by a measurement.

Pre-Experimental Designs

The primary way in which the so-called pre-experimental designs differ from true experiments is in their lack of randomization. Because of this lack, technically pre-experimental designs represent quasi-experimental research. These designs are examined here because they are occasionally employed in research, and because they serve as the basis for true experimental designs.

A second important distinction between experimental and pre-experimental designs results from the above-mentioned differences in their use of randomization. All pre-experimental designs share the weakness of being open to one or more of the threats to internal validity discussed in Chapter 3. True experimental designs are not vulnerable to internal validity threats.

The first pre-experimental design was labeled by Campbell and Stanley (1963) 'The One-Shot Case Study.' Subjects are chosen through some method other than randomization, exposed to a form of treatment, then observed.

$$X \qquad O$$

Because no measures are taken before treatment, it is quite difficult for the researcher employing this design to credibly claim treatment effectiveness. The researcher has no baseline measure of the sample or reason to believe the sample is typical of the population, so questions about the internal and external validity of the study abound. The primary threat to external validity is the interaction of selection and treatment. Indeed this design is so severely flawed as to render it essentially useless.

The second pre-experimental design improves slightly on the first by including a pre-treatment observation. This design, therefore, does enable the experimenter to demonstrate change in the experimental group. There is still no control group or alternative treatment group, however, so it is still hard to claim that the change was due to the treatment.

$$O \qquad X \qquad O$$

This design is vulnerable to the threats to internal validity posed by history, maturation, testing, instrumentation, and the interactions involving selection. Threats to external validity include the interactions of testing and selection with treatment.

The third pre-experimental design employs two groups of subjects. The first group receives treatment, then is observed. The second group is not treated but is observed at the same time as the first group.

$$X \qquad O \qquad \text{Group 1}$$
$$O \qquad \text{Group 2}$$

This comparison weakens the potential argument that observed changes would have come without treatment. Because of the lack of randomization and any pre-treatment measures, this design shares many of the weaknesses of the one-shot case study. Selection, mortality, and the selection–maturation interaction represent threats to internal validity; selection–treatment interaction threatens external validity.

In summary, all three designs are so seriously flawed that their use should be avoided whenever possible. As we will soon see, introducing randomization procedures into essentially these same designs effectively eliminates threats to internal validity and substantially improves the designs.

True Experimental Designs

In all three true experimental designs, subjects are chosen through random sampling procedures. In each design there are also control or alternative treatment groups on which comparisons can be based. This combination eliminates threats to internal validity for these designs.

The first true experimental design compares a treatment with a control group.

R	O	X	O	Group 1
R	O		O	Group 2

Subjects for both are chosen using randomization techniques, both groups are pre-tested, the treatment is administered to one group, and both groups are remeasured. The initial equivalence of the groups can be established, and changes in the treatment group that do not appear in the control group can plausibly be assigned to the treatment. The primary threat to external validity lies in the interaction of the treatment and testing. Campbell and Stanley have questioned the extent to which the threat of selection by treatment interaction can be controlled in any true experimental design and have pointed out the possibility of reactive arrangements (situations in which these undesirable interactions occur). However, to a certain extent the size of the effect of the interactions can be assessed statistically.

The second true experimental design is a variation of the final pre-experimental design that includes randomization.

R	X	O	Group 1
R		O	Group 2

Subjects are not pre-tested, and therefore equivalence cannot be directly demonstrated. However, the researcher can somewhat safely assume equivalence based on randomization (given a large enough number of subjects in each group) and need not be concerned about the possibility that pre-testing is interacting with the treatment.

The final true experimental design was designed by Solomon (1949) and is known as the Solomon Four Group Design.

R	O	X	O	Group 1
R	O		O	Group 2
R		X	O	Group 3
R			O	Group 4

The four groups of this design eliminate the problems we noted with the pre-experimental pre- and post-test design. Randomization procedures are used to construct all groups. The first group assesses change with treatment. The second group controls for the possibility of change without treatment. The third group controls for the possibility that the pre-testing influences response to treatment. And the fourth group assesses an initially theoretically equivalent group without any experimental intervention. If, following treatment, effects appear that differentiate groups 1 and 3 from groups 2 and 4, it is difficult to generate plausible explanations for them other than the treatment.

If you will glance back at the true experimental designs you may be struck by the fact that the first two designs represent the two halves of the Solomon Four Group Design. Because this design counters so many alternative explanations for results it represents the strongest design. It must be pointed out, though, that any one of the true experimental designs enables better research than any of the pre-experimental designs. Perfect random sampling is, of course, not always possible. But the adoption of some form of probability sampling increases the strength of research so much that such methods should be adopted whenever possible.

□ DISADVANTAGES OF TRUE EXPERIMENTS □

Although in most cases the true experiment should be the design of choice, there are some circumstances that prevent its use. Some of these situations arise in both laboratory and field experiments, others are more commonly encountered in field experiments.

The first difficulty was alluded to in the discussion of variables in Chapter 2. When the phenomenon of interest is a single attribute variable, it is not possible to randomize group membership. (Recall that an attribute variable represents subjects' characteristics such as age and is therefore not manipulable.) The use of a single, nonrandom, nonmanipulable independent variable alters the character of the research from true experimental to non-experimental form.

A second disadvantage of true experimental design lies in the amount of time often necessary to conduct true experimental research. It is not uncommon for a true experimental study to take several painstaking years to complete. If experimental results are to be the basis of policy decisions and results are needed more rapidly, it is often preferable to use a quasi-experimental or non-experimental design to capitalize on natural variability of the independent variable of interest.

There are situations in which it would be unethical to manipulate the independent variable. Early research on lung cancer and cigarette smoking made use of archival information on the rate of smoking of lung cancer patients. Clearly it would have been medically unethical to set up a true experiment where the goal of treatment was to cause a life-threatening disease. Similarly, a researcher would not test a potentially teratogenic drug on expectant mothers. In such cases non-experimental research is the only ethical alternative.

Because true experimental designs by definition involve providing treatment to some subjects and withholding it from others, access to samples may become a problem, particularly in field settings. Health care administrators may not allow permission for the conduct of true experiments while allowing quasi-experimental or non-experimental research to proceed.

It is often particularly problematical to employ true experimental designs in field settings. It takes a particularly clever and creative researcher to overcome the control problems presented by natural settings. As noted by Cook and Campbell (1979, p 385): "The desirability of randomized experiments in field settings is less in question than their feasibility."

Two of the disadvantages of the use of true experiments in field settings involve the control group. The first consideration is the ethical question posed by withholding treatment from the control group. If the experimenter believes the treatment to be effective, it becomes difficult ethically to justify non-treatment of control subjects. This problem is often circumvented through the modification of the control group procedure discussed previously. Instead of receiving no treatment, the control group either receives an alternative treatment of approximately equal desirability or is treated in the usual manner for such cases. Because it can be argued that subjects are receiving treatment at least as effective as the norm, the ethical problems are reduced.

The second disadvantage related to the use of control groups is closely connected with the first. Even when the experimental design allows for the use of a no-treatment control, the experimenter must monitor the control group closely. In many cases, more is going on in the control group than planned for (or desired by) the experimenter. Several potential problems were alluded to in the discussion of validity. Subjects may hear of alternative treatments that appear more desirable and react by becoming either competitive or apathetic. If subjects are not receiving treatment they may become resentful, which leads to our final disadvantage of the use of true experiments in field settings.

Resentful subjects may choose to drop out of research studies. Such resentment is probably particularly likely to appear in subjects in a control group (either no-treatment or alternative-treatment). Differential attrition rates across conditions may jeopardize randomization of groups and introduce systematic bias. At the beginning of the study, when informed consent is being sought from potential subjects, it is wise for the researcher to be as candid as the design allows about possible treatments the subject may receive and to obtain consent before assigning the subject to a condition. If subjects are aware that they may be assigned to a less desirable condition but agree to participate anyway, they may be less likely to leave the study.

□ SITUATIONS CONDUCIVE TO TRUE EXPERIMENTS □

Fortunately, there exist a number of situations in which the use of true experimental designs is facilitated. In these situations randomization either is not a problem or is actually an advantage.

There are some situations in the real world in which the randomization associated with lotteries is entirely accepted, even expected; for example, the assignment of college students to dormitory rooms and the use of lotteries for policy purposes. As mentioned earlier in this chapter, when demand outstrips supply, randomization often represents the "fairest," most ethical allocation of the resource. In this case randomization is perceived by subjects as a positive characteristic (as long as the assignment procedure is perceived as truly equitable). Randomization also has an appeal in the opposite case, in which subjects do not express a preference as to their assignment. Here again, randomization is perceived as acceptable.

The final pair of situations conducive to the use of true experiments involves cases in which the need for change is clearly recognized. When change is mandated, but the content or structure of the optimal change is unclear, an experiment may be welcomed as a means of acquiring desirable information. Even when there is some particular innovation to be introduced, in situations where all units to be eventually affected cannot be serviced at once, an experiment may be employed to assess the effectiveness of the innovation in the units where change is implemented earlier.

The use of true experimental designs, with their characteristics of manipulation, control, and randomization, provides the researcher with his or her most powerful tool and most convincing results. Often the employment of such designs calls on the ingenuity and creativity of the researcher, particularly in field settings. The advantages to be accrued from the additional time and thought necessary to implement these designs, however, usually represent a more than adequate return on investment.

□ SUMMARY □

True experiments are characterized by manipulation, control, and randomization. Pre-experimental designs lack randomization, quasi-experimental designs lack either control or randomization, and non-experimental research lacks manipulation. True experimental designs provide maximum safeguard against threats to validity and reliability. Use of the other designs allows for various alternative explanations for results.

True experiments may be conducted either in the laboratory or in the field (natural environment). Although laboratory conditions assist in control procedures, field settings are more likely to approximate "real-life" conditions. Therefore, although internal validity may be superior in laboratory research, external validity is likely to be superior for field experiments.

□ KEY TERMS □

experiment

quasi-experiment

non-experiment

manipulation

control

bias

field experiment

laboratory experiment

control group

□□ 5 □□

Quasi-Experimental Designs

- □ *Non-Equivalent Control Group Designs*
  - □ *Untreated Control Group with Pre- and Post-Test*
  - □ *Untreated Control Group with Proxy Pre-Test Measures*
  - □ *Untreated Control Group with Separate Pre-Test and Post-Test Samples*
  - □ *Untreated Control Group with Pre-Test Measures at More Than One Point in Time*
  - □ *Reversed Treatment Non-Equivalent Control Group with Pre- and Post-Test*
- □ *Designs Employing the Subjects as Their Own Control Group*
  - □ *Non-Equivalent Dependent Variables Design*
  - □ *Removed Treatment with Pre- and Post-Testing*
  - □ *Repeated-Treatment Design*
- □ *Cohort Designs*
  - □ *Institutional Cycles Design*
  - □ *Recurrent Institutional Cycles Design*
- □ *Regression-Discontinuity Designs*
- □ *Interrupted Time Series Designs*
- □ *Disadvantages and Advantages of Quasi-Experimental Designs*

69

Often in the real world—and especially in applied research in the field—it is simply not possible to conduct research employing true experimental designs. When the difficulty encountered involves either randomization or control, quasi-experimental designs should be used instead. These designs represent the next level of rigor in the hierarchy of research designs. In this chapter we will examine five categories of quasi-experimental designs: (1) designs employing non-equivalent control groups, (2) designs in which the subjects are used as their own control group, (3) cohort designs, (4) regression-discontinuity designs, and (5) interrupted time series designs. These designs and the discussion to follow are drawn from the work of Cook and Campbell (1979). For each type of design we will consider the various threats to internal validity to which the designs are most vulnerable and the pattern of results that can most readily be interpreted (that is, the pattern that allows us to consider our treatment effective).

□ NON-EQUIVALENT CONTROL GROUP DESIGNS □

The non-equivalent control group designs share in common the fact that subjects are not chosen or assigned in a random manner. In these cases it is unsafe to assume that the treatment and control groups are similar—hence the name. This difficulty renders all five designs of this type particularly vulnerable to four of the threats to internal validity: (1) selection by history interaction, (2) instrumentation, (3) selection by maturation interaction, and 4) statistical regression.

Untreated Control Group with Pre- and Post-Test

The most commonly employed non-equivalent control group design involves pre- and post-testing for both the experimental and control groups, with only the experimental group receiving treatment. Conceptually what we are interested in examining is the extent of difference between these two observations or sets of scores.

$$O \quad X \quad O \qquad \text{Group 1 (treatment)}$$
$$O \qquad\quad\; O \qquad \text{Group 2 (control)}$$

According to Cook and Campbell (1979), as will be discussed in Chapter 13, statistical analysis of the difference in scores is conceptually the phenomenon of interest rather than the analysis of the gain or loss scores.

The results of this type of design fall into five characteristic patterns which we will employ to discuss the most serious threats to internal validity. Understand that more than one of the threats can be invoked to explain each pattern. We are only using one per design to illustrate possible alternative explanations. The first pattern involves no change in scores for the control group with the treatment group showing a decrement pre- to post-test.

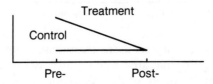

Although it would be nice to assume this pattern resulted from an effective treatment, a plausible rival interpretation involves the selection by history interaction. This is also sometimes referred to as a local history effect. If, as often occurs, subjects in the treatment group are drawn from one hospital and controls from another, any sort of occurrence in one site that may affect subjects may well not occur in the other site. Thus any apparent gain in scores could represent an artifact, not a true effect of treatment.

In a second commonly encountered pattern of results for this type of study, both the control and treatment groups show pre- to post-test gains, but at different rates—that is, the slopes of the lines differ. It is unfortunately true that such a pattern could result from instrumentation effects. Since the two groups begin at different levels of the dependent measure, an instrument whose sensitivity is not uniform throughout the measurement range may be more sensitive to changes in one group's scores than to changes in the other's.

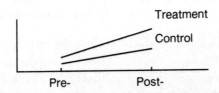

The two groups' rates of change may in fact be the same, but the instrument would make it appear otherwise. An analogy would be a thermometer that responds sensitively to changes of one degree at temperatures between 80 and 90 degrees but only responds to changes of three degrees or more at temperatures between 120 and 130 degrees.

The third pattern of results vulnerable to interpretations not involving the treatment under investigation is one in which the control group's scores again show no change pre- to post-testing, but the treatment group's scores show a pre- to post-test gain. A selection by maturation interaction might be expected to result in just such a pattern.

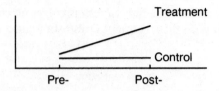

In such an interaction, subjects in the treatment group exhibit changes in the dependent measure that are based on increases in age, or strength, or practice and are independent of the treatment. Because the groups were not equivalent to begin with, subjects in the control group do not exhibit the same maturational changes.

The final pattern of results is vulnerable to explanation based on statistical regression. In this pattern, scores for the treatment group are lower than those of controls on the pre-test, but by the post-test period have risen to meet the control group's scores.

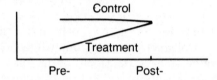

As you will recall from the discussion in Chapter 3, atypically high or low scores on a measure are expected to move in the direction of the "average" score. If the control group initially scored primarily in the moderate range we would not expect to see a great difference in post-test scores. If, however, the treatment group generally scored quite low on pre-test measures we would expect to see post-test gains entirely independent of treatment.

Before you abandon all hope of ever claiming treatment effectiveness for the results of a non-equivalent control group design, let us hasten to point out that there is a pattern of results that can be most plausibly interpreted as due to the experimental treatment. In this pattern, the control group's scores are higher than the treatment group's on the pre-test.

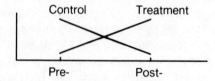

By the post-test, however, the treatment group's scores are significantly higher than the control group's.

The selection interactions do not provide plausible explanations because we would have to see offsetting historical events having opposite effects or maturational trends in opposite directions. Instrumentation cannot plausibly be used as an explanation because both groups have moved through the same range of scores—thus both theoretically have been affected by any weaknesses in the instrument's sensitivity. Regression could be used to explain scores moving closer to each other in value but cannot explain the reversal in this pattern.

Clearly, then, this pattern of results is by far the most desirable and useful for researchers to demonstrate the effectiveness of treatments. This is not to say that treatment effects may not exist in results exhibiting one of the other patterns. It is simply to say that when this pattern is found, the rival explanations for results to which the other patterns are vulnerable can more easily and more safely be dismissed.

Untreated Control Group with Proxy Pre-test Measures

In research designs using an untreated control group and proxy pre-test measures, we again see pre- and post-testing in treatment and control groups chosen in a non-random manner, with the treatment group receiving the experimental manipulation.

O_{A1}	X	O_{B2}	Group 1 (treatment)
O_{A1}		O_{B2}	Group 2 (control)

The primary difference lies in the measures used at the pre- and post-test observation points. Whereas in the first design the same measures were employed at both measurement points, in this design different instruments are utilized.

The results of studies employing this design are quite difficult to interpret. The correlation between the proxy pre-test measure and the post-test measure is almost always lower than the correlation between pre- and post-test scores on the same measure. Given this lower correlation the reliability of measurement may serve as a plausible explanation for results.

The ideal pattern of results from the point of view of treatment effects occurs when the two groups' scores are similar on the pre-test measure, the scores between groups on the post-treatment measure are significantly different, and there exists a strong correlation between scores for the two measures (high reliability), as seen below.

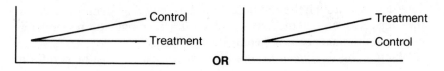

If the two groups differ greatly on the pre-test measures, statistical tests to compensate for these differences generally provide insufficient adjustment and thus are likely to indicate a treatment effect when in fact post-test group differences stem from the groups' initial nonequivalence.

If there are very small post-test differences between the treatment and control groups and the correlation between the two measures is low, the tendency will be to assign this lack of difference to a lack of treatment effects when in fact the measurement may be failing to detect effects that actually exist because its reliability is low.

Why, then, would anyone employ such a design? In several situations this design is useful. When the phenomenon of interest is susceptible to practice effects or when subjects develop skills in taking the pre-test, it is desirable to employ related but different pre- and post-test measures. Also, when the post-measure involves skills that the subject was expected to acquire from the treatment (e.g., a training program of some type) and was not expected to possess at the time of the pre-test observation, measurement of a similar ability is the researcher's only recourse. (Note that we don't dispense entirely with a pre-test because our ability to demonstrate similarity between the groups before the administration of treatment considerably strengthens the case for post-treatment differences being the result of the treatment.)

Untreated Control Group with Separate Pre-Test and Post-Test Samples

If concerned about the effects of testing on subjects, a researcher may choose a design using an untreated control group with separate pre-test and post-test samples, employing different samples of subjects at each measurement point. (The vertical dotted line indicates a change in subjects.)

0	⋮	X	0	Group 1 (treatment)
0	⋮		0	Group 2 (control)

Given our concern all along with the equivalence of our treatment and control groups, doesn't the use of four rather than two groups exacerbate this problem? Absolutely. For this reason this design can be stengthened considerably through the addition of randomization procedures in choosing subjects for each of the four samples (which removes this research format from the category of nonequivalent designs!)

When using this weak design, the experimenter must be careful to check scores to determine not only that the treatment and control groups are equivalent at the beginning of the study, and that the pre- and post-treatment samples within both the treatment condition and the control condition are equivalent, but also that the second treatment and control samples are equivalent on any characteristics that might influence treatment outcome. If an experimenter must employ this design, great care must be taken with sampling. If all of the above mentioned equivalences between sample groups can be demonstrated and only the treatment condition exhibits pre- and post-treatment changes then treatment effectiveness can be argued.

Untreated Control Group with Pretest Measures at More Than One Point in Time

A design using an untreated control group with pretest measures at more than one point in time takes two pre-treatment measures on both the experimental and control groups. This duplication of pre-testing provides the experimenter with potentially very valuable information.

$$O_1 \quad O_2 \quad X \quad O_3 \qquad \text{Group 1 (treatment)}$$
$$O_1 \quad O_2 \qquad O_3 \qquad \text{Group 2 (control)}$$

Having two pretest measures allows a check of maturational rates between conditions. If the rates are the same before the intervention, a change for only the experimental group points to treatment effects and seriously weakens an argument in favor of a selection by maturation interaction.

The two pre-measures will also help to identify whether an observation period is atypical. If pre-test measures differ radically within one group, something unusual may have influenced scores at one of the points. Clearly a researcher would not wish to base comparisons on a noncomparable point. Again, the researcher would like to obtain results in which the pre-test scores for both groups are consistent within and between conditions, and where only the treatment group shows change across the O_2 to O_3 interval.

If this design is so strong, why is it not seen more often? One possible reason involves the necessity to obtain permission from funding agencies or administrators who control access to subjects. These, unfortunately, are likely to balk at the additional time and effort involved in a seemingly redundant pre-test. When time and access allow, however, this design is one of the strongest (in terms of research design) of the non-equivalent control group designs.

Reversed Treatment Non-Equivalent Control Group
With Pre- and Post-Test

In designs using a reversed treatment non-equivalent control group with pre- and post-test, both groups receive an experimental manipulation. The "treatment" group receives the experimental manipulation while the "control" group receives a treatment believed by the researcher to reverse the effects of treatment.

0	X+	0	Group 1 (treatment)
0	X—	0	Group 2 (control)

Clearly for health sciences research aimed at providing evidence of the effectiveness of treatment it is ethically unthinkable to deliberately do harm to a patient. However, in research of a more phenomenological nature within the profession (e.g., attitudes of practitioners) such designs may have a place. In defense of the design it must be stated that such studies are often particularly strong in terms of construct validity since a construct must be very tightly defined in order to define its opposite.

□ DESIGNS EMPLOYING THE SUBJECTS □
AS THEIR OWN CONTROL GROUP

In this second group of designs, in which subjects are employed as controls, we no longer see separate treatment and control groups. Control is enhanced by virtue of the fact that (as mentioned in Chapter 3) such repeated-measures designs help reduce the amount of random noise based on subject characteristics. It is safe to assume that characteristics such as age, gender, temperament, and intelligence will not vary much over the course of a study. Using subjects as their own control group provides the researcher with the most equivalent control group possible .

However, the fact that subjects receive more than one treatment increases the problem of testing or reactivity effects. The inability to compare results with an untreated group may weaken inferences about observed changes. For these reasons (and the lack of randomization procedures) these designs remain quasi-experimental in nature.

Non-Equivalent Dependent Variables Design

In non-equivalent dependent-variables designs subjects are pre- and post-tested using more than one dependent measure—labeled in the diagram as A and B.

$$O_{1AB} \quad X \quad O_{2AB}$$

Measure A is the variable of interest in the study and it is expected the measure will change with the treatment. Measure B is a conceptually similar measure that is not expected to be altered by the experimental manipulation.

In its pure form as diagrammed above, this design is considered by Cook and Campbell (1979) to be one of the weaker designs in terms of successfully defending against alternative explanations for results. The desired pattern of results—a change in Measure A and no change in Measure B across the treatment interval—is open to plausible alternative explanations. The design can be strengthened through the use of multiple measures and the addition of supplemental pre- and post-test measurement points. As discussed above, additional measurement points aid in assessing the typicality of measurement points and any maturational changes that may occur independent of the treatment.

Removed Treatment with Pre- and Post-Testing

In the health sciences, where most treatments are intended to demonstrate long-term effects or cures, designs using removed treatment with pre- and post-testing, which first pre- and post-test subjects across a treatment interval then repeat the pre- and post-testing across an interval in which the treatment has been removed, may not be particularly useful.

$$O_1 \quad X \quad O_2 \qquad O_3 \quad \overline{X} \quad O_4$$

In addition to practical problems in removing a treatment there may be serious ethical problems in removing a treatment when doing so may harm the well-being of a patient. Removing the treatment may also cause resentment and noncooperation in the subjects, which could well obscure effects of the treatment.

If this design is to be employed, the researcher must ensure that all the time intervals are equal. Otherwise the clearest pattern of results—gains across the first interval and losses across the second interval—may be explained away because subjects simply had more time to change during one of the intervals. Unfortunately, in this design the effects of a treatment that is effective for a long period may be underestimated, since gains that appear in the treatment interval can be sustained throughout the interval in which treatment is removed.

Repeated-Treatment Design

In repeated-treatment designs, treatment is introduced, removed, and reintroduced. As in the design just discussed, this design is only useful when treatment effects are believed to be short-lived.

$$O_1 \quad X \quad O_2 \quad \overline{X} \quad O_3 \quad X \quad O_4$$

An additional requirement for this design is that treatment effects should not be additive or reactive with earlier treatment effects. The ideally interpretable pattern of effects would exhibit gains in measures between O_1 and O_2 and between O_3 and O_4 with a drop in scores across the O_2-O_3 interval.

In many studies it is desirable to keep subjects unaware of research hypotheses. (The reasons for this will be discussed in Chapter 9.) This design makes it particularly difficult to keep subjects naive. Results may be explained by the subjects' guessing the research hypothesis and responding according to what they perceive as the researcher's desires (demand effects).

□ COHORT DESIGNS □

In cohort designs, we again see the use of a comparison group to aid in interpreting changes in the treatment group. However, the groups are not observed or evaluated at the same time. Cook and Campbell (1979, p. 127) define cohorts as "groups of respondents who follow each other through formal institutions or informal institutions like the family." Thus, if research were to be conducted on your class in research design, the control cohort might be either last semester's or next semester's class at your institution (or both). Although obviously not randomly chosen (and therefore not as comparable as randomly chosen samples), cohorts are likely to be fairly comparable with each other to the extent that entrance or retention requirements of institutions tend to result in a fairly homogeneous group of people. Another advantage of cohort designs is the probable availability of records kept by the institution. Hospital or school records may provide the necessary information on the untreated cohort.

The basic cohort design involves examination of records or measurements of one group and subsequent treatment and then measurement of a later cohort. The shift to the right for Group 2 indicates this difference in time frame and the wavy line separating the groups indicates the use of cohorts.

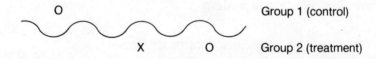

This design is quite weak in defending against alternative explanations for results provided by threats to internal validity. Because of the difference in the time of the observations, history may provide a strong rival explanation for results. Without any direct measures to assess equivalence of the cohorts, selection may prove a factor in results. For example, if your institution were to require a course in research design initially at the freshman level then changed the curriculum to move the course to the senior year, a study using one class immediately before the change and one immediately after the change would clearly have subjects who differed on a number of characeristics that might affect the study's measures.

Another weakness of the basic cohort design is that it ignores the possibility that subjects in the treated cohort may receive different amounts of treatment. To expand the example above, suppose the treatment under examination was the introduction of a new teaching technique in courses on research design. Scores on a comprehensive final examination from a course employing the old techniques would be compared with scores on the same exam achieved by the treated class.

While in most institutions most students are conscientious and attend class regularly, there are usually some students who do not attend class. If a student only attended 10% of the class lectures that employed the new teaching techniques, we would not expect to see an effect of the techniques as clearly as we would expect to see it in a student with perfect attendance.

When it is possible to differentiate levels of treatment received within the experimental cohort, the basic cohort design can be strengthened by considering these levels separately as diagrammed, where the subscripts on the X's indicate separate levels of treatment.

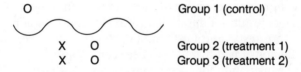

O			Group 1 (control)
X	O		Group 2 (treatment 1)
X	O		Group 3 (treatment 2)

If stronger effects are seen for the group receiving more of the treatment, arguments for the effectiveness of the treatment are enhanced. Such results also help rule out an explanation based on testing effects because all levels of the treatment group would be expected to demonstrate such effects.

Institutional Cycles Design

When it is not possible to stratify levels of treatment, the basic cohort design can still be strengthened through the use of multiple measurement points. Cook and Campbell (1979) have called this the Institutional Cycles Design. The additional measurement points help to reduce the strength of arguments based on maturation of subjects.

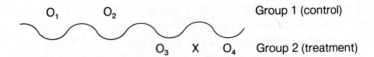

This design is commonly employed in organizations and can be strengthened even further through the use of several untreated comparison cohorts. The use of several comparison groups with comparable patterns across the measurement interval helps to eliminate historically based alternative explanations because events with similar effects on the research measurements would have to have occurred for each group.

Recurrent Institutional Cycles Design

The final cohort design is known as the recurrent institutional cycles design (Campbell & Stanley, 1963). In this design three cohorts are employed. The first receives the treatment and a post-test only. The second receives the more usual pre-test, treatment, post-test sequence

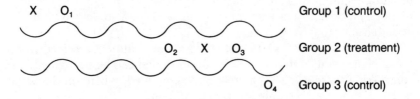

The third cohort receives only a pre-test at the beginning of the cycle. The ideal pattern of results for this design would involve comparable scores for O_2 and O_4 (pre-tests) and for O_1 and O_3 (post-tests). Treatment effects would be demonstrated by changes between O_2 and O_3. History is again an unlikely explanation for such results as historical events with equivalent effects would have to be recurrent.

□ REGRESSION-DISCONTINUITY DESIGNS □

Regression-discontinuity designs differ from the designs we have considered thus far in that assignment to groups is based on scores obtained on some pre-treatment measure. Subjects who fall below a cut-off point on the variable, such as income or resources available, are provided with the treatment (e.g., a training program or supplemental services) because of their early disadvantaged status. On post-testing (after treatment), scores for the treatment group would be expected to exhibit change while those for the untreated group would be expected to remain static.

Individual scores are plotted on a graph using the horizontal axis for pre-test scores and the vertical axis for post-test scores as shown (after Cook and Campbell, 1979).

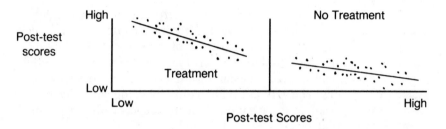

Through a technique known as linear regression (discussed in Chapter 13), equations are derived that describe lines that best fit the pattern shown by the plotted points. If the treatment is effective the lines for the treatment and control groups should be discontinuous—that is, the line should break at the cut-off point—thus the name, regression-discontinuity design. Because of the manner of assignment to condition, selection, and the selection by maturation and selection by instrumentation innteractions may provide strong rival explanations for results.

□ INTERRUPTED TIME SERIES DESIGNS □

Time series designs involve taking measures over an extended period. There are two types of time series designs—one that qualifies as quasi-experimental research and will be discussed here, and another that is an example of non-experimental research and will be discussed in Chapter 6.

Designs of the first type are known as interrupted time series designs and involve an experimental intervention at some point in the measurement series. Measurements subsequent to the intervention seek to assess the impact of the treatment. The other type of design is known simply as time series. It qualifies as non-experimental research because there is no manipulation. Measurements are taken to assess naturally occurring variation with the intent to forecast future events.

Interrupted time series designs are a useful alternative for the researcher who wishes to examine whether treatment affects the rate of change in a phenomenon that is itself expected to evidence change (e.g., whether treatment increases the rate at which patients regain mobility after breaking a leg). These designs may also prove useful in assessing the permanence of change following treatment, since in several designs the treatment is only administered during one of the measurement intervals while measures continue to be taken several times post-treatment.

The major rival alternative explanation for results for single-intervention designs is history. It may be difficult to refute arguments that treatment results are due to an extraneous event that occurred while treatment was being administered.

Instrumentation is a threat to all of the interrupted time series designs in that they usually depend on archival records for their data. Record-keeping procedures may change in the course of the study. The definition of terms may change (the definition of a term such as *depression*, for example, may broaden), causing the types and numbers of cases to alter in later stages of the study. The very fact that records are being employed as data in a study may result in sensitization of record keepers with a resultant alteration in methods.

A final problem associated with interrupted time series data is the existence of seasonal or cyclical variations based on factors other than the experimental manipulation. For example, a study of the effectiveness of a public awareness campaign on the value of wearing seat belts that used counts of automobile injuries over a one-year period would have to correct for seasonal variations in the sheer numbers of automobiles on the road at any point in time. Fortunately there are statistical procedures available that help remove such irrelevant variation.

The basic form of the interrupted time series design involves multiple pre-test measurement points, a single interval of intervention, and multiple post-treatment measurements.

$$O_1 \quad O_2 \quad O_3 \quad O_4 \quad O_5 X O_6 \quad O_7 \quad O_8 \quad O_9 \quad O_{10}$$

As mentioned above, the threat of history is particularly severe for this design. To counter this problem, the use of a control group (for whom records are maintained but to whom no treatment is administered) is of considerable assistance.

$$O_1 \quad O_2 \quad O_3 \quad O_4 \quad O_5 X O_6 \quad O_7 \quad O_8 \quad O_9 \quad O_{10} \qquad \text{Group 1}$$
$$O_1 \quad O_2 \quad O_3 \quad O_4 \quad O_5 \quad O_6 \quad O_7 \quad O_8 \quad O_9 \quad O_{10} \qquad \text{Group 2}$$

For all interrupted time series designs, intervals should be of equal length. The control group would also be susceptible to any history effects, so the ability to show that these effects are absent in the control group strengthens the design.

The threat of a history-based alternative explanation is further weakened by another variation on the basic design.

$$O_1 \quad O_2 \quad O_3 X O_4 \quad O_5 \quad O_6 \quad O_7 \quad O_8 \quad O_9 \quad O_{10} \quad O_{11} \qquad \text{Group 1}$$
$$O_1 \quad O_2 \quad O_3 \quad O_4 \quad O_5 \quad O_6 \quad O_7 \quad O_8 X O_9 \quad O_{10} \quad O_{11} \qquad \text{Group 2}$$

The first group receives the treatment in the interval between O_3 and O_4. The second group receives the same intervention but not until the interval between O_8 and O_9. In effect the two groups alternate in being the control group for the other group. Because measurement points occur at the same times for the groups, history effects should appear in and affect both groups.

The final interrupted time series design involving a single intervention point employs non-equivalent dependent variables as measures for a treatment and control group.

$$O_{A1} \quad O_{A2} \quad O_{A3} \quad O_{A4} \quad O_{A5} X O_{A6} \quad O_{A7} \quad O_{A8} \quad O_{A9} \quad O_{A10} \qquad \text{Group 1}$$
$$O_{B1} \quad O_{B2} \quad O_{B3} \quad O_{B4} \quad O_{B5} X O_{B6} \quad O_{B7} \quad O_{B8} \quad O_{B9} \quad O_{B10} \qquad \text{Group 2}$$

The two measures should be conceptually similar yet sufficiently disparate that the treatment is expected to affect the measure for one group but not the other. This design variation also enhances construct validity by tightening the focus of the treatment.

The final two variations of the interrupted time series design involve both the administration and the removal of treatment from subjects. Thus they share all of the ethical and practical problems discussed previously in relation to removal of treatment. The major advantage associated with these two designs is that treatment is not administered during only a single observation interval. This feature may be especially useful in investigations of treatments in which delays can be expected before effects are noted.

In the interrupted time series design with removal of treatment, subjects are observed for five measurement intervals, treatment is administered between intervals O_5 and O_9, then treatment is removed and observations continue to O_{13}. As mentioned, this design is especially suited for slow-acting treatments.

$$O_1 \quad O_2 \quad O_3 \quad O_4 \quad O_5 X O_6 X O_7 X O_8 X O_9 \, \overline{X} O_{10} \quad O_{11} \quad O_{12} \quad O_{13}$$

After removal of treatment the repeated observations allow the researcher to determine the longevity of treatment effects.

History is basically eliminated as an explanation for results because an event that caused results in intervals O_5 to O_8 would have to reverse itself for intervals O_9 to O_{13}.

If, however, measurements showed change during the treatment period that was maintained afterward, it would be difficult to determine whether this change reflected a long-lasting treatment effect or a long-lasting historical effect. Another concern must be the reaction of subjects to this design. Losses in scores during the final phase of the study may be explained as resentful demoralization on the part of subjects.

The final variation of the interrupted time series design can only be utilized for treatments that are very short-lived (and is therefore probably inappropriate for most health sciences research).

$$O_1 \quad O_2XO_3 \quad O_4\overline{X}O_5 \quad O_6XO_7 \quad O_8\overline{X}O_9 \quad O_{10}XO_{11} \quad O_{12}\overline{X}O_{13} \quad O_{14}$$

The design involves an initial observation period, then periods of alternatively providing and removing treatment, then a final observation point. Control is difficult for this design and the reactions of subjects may present serious problems. This design is often utilized in the behavioral sciences for behavior modification programs.

□ DISADVANTAGES AND ADVANTAGES □ OF QUASI-EXPERIMENTAL DESIGNS

As should be clear from the discussions of the individual designs in this chapter, the use of quasi-experimental designs is fraught with disadvantages, which fall into three categories. The first disadvantage involves validity problems in explaining results. All of the designs are vulnerable to various threats to internal validity and many also have problems of construct validity. The second category of disadvantage involves the practical implementation of a number of the designs. It is questionable whether some health science treatments that lead to cure or alleviation of a condition can be removed, and unfortunately the stronger studies in terms of withstanding internal validity threats often involve removal of treatment. Finally, and most seriously, there are ethical issues involved with the use of some of the designs. Beyond the question of whether treatment effects can be removed is the question of whether it is ethical to do so. Even more ethically inappropriate would be the adoption of a design that would deliberately worsen a patient's condition through the reversal of a treatment effect.

There are, however, advantages associated with the judicious and ethical use of quasi-experimental designs. In many field settings, quasi-experimental designs are far more practical and feasible than true experiments—which may simply be impossible to implement. Permission allowing access to subjects may be denied to true experimental studies but may be forthcoming for quasi-experiments.

The final, and greatest, advantage of quasi-experimental designs involves external validity. Because most quasi-experimental studies are performed in field settings, with all of the concomitant noise and lack of control inherent in such settings, the results of these studies are often more generalizable than those of true experiments. A high level of external validity is a particular bonus to the researcher in the applied health sciences who, because of practical constraints, is often forced to employ this type of design.

□ SUMMARY □

Quasi-experimental research designs can be categorized into five groups: (1) designs employing non-equivalent control groups, (2) designs in which subjects are used as their own control group, (3) cohort designs, (4) regression-discontinuity designs, and (5) interrupted time series designs. Because all quasi-experimental designs lack some of the characteristics of true experimental designs, all are vulnerable to threats to internal validity and some are vulnerable to threats to construct validity. In addition, there are practical and ethical constraints on the use of such designs in health-science research.

Advantages of quasi-experimental designs include ease of use in field settings where strict control is impossible, and strong external validity.

□ KEY TERMS □

non-equivalent control groups   cohort
proxy pre-tests   regression-discontinuity

□□ 6 □□

Non-Experimental Research Designs

The final major category of research designs, the non-experimental designs, all lack any manipulation of the independent variable by the experimenter. Instead, both the independent and dependent variables are observed and measured. There are several reasons why these designs might be employed although they are the weakest of research designs. In cases where the independent variable of interest is an attribute such as age or diagnosis, manipulation is clearly not possible. In other cases manipulation is not performed for ethical reasons. Investigators interested in the type of head injuries most commonly sustained in high-speed head-on collisions obviously cannot involve subjects in staging such collisions. Thus the non-experimental designs occupy an important place in the hierarchy of research designs.

Non-experimental designs can be classified into two basic categories: ex post facto research and descriptive research. Even though no manipulations or interventions are performed, the intent of ex post facto research is to explore the relationships between variables. Descriptive research, as the name implies, is more commonly concerned with observing and documenting phenomena.

□ EX POST FACTO RESEARCH □

As mentioned above, ex post facto research seeks to describe the relationships between variables. Kerlinger (1965, p 379)) defines ex post facto research as "systematic empirical inquiry in which the scientist does not have direct control of independent variables because their manifestations have already occurred or because they are inherently not amenable to manipulation. Inferences about relations among variables are made, without direct intervention, from concomitant variation of independent and dependent variables." Although we will consider retrospective and prospective sub-categories of this type of research, both of these can be considered to be what is known as correlational research. A correlation measures the extent of the covariation between two variables. As is discussed in Chapter 13, there are several statistical techniques that quantify the extent of the relationship. Because there has been no manipulation of variables, evidence of a strong relationship tells us only that a relationship exists. It tells us nothing about the underlying causes of the relationship. Inferring causation from a correlation is an error too commonly encountered in the research literature.

Retrospective Studies

In retrospective studies the researcher begins with an effect and looks back to try to identify the cause. Epidemiologic studies are often of this kind. The researcher first identifies an effect and then collects data from subjects (or archives) on behaviors. An example of this type of research was the case involving the medication Thalidomide. When women began giving birth to children with an unusual and very distinctive malformation of the limbs, extensive research on the mothers' behaviors during pregnancy identified the drug as a common factor. Note that such evidence technically does not prove causation. Laboratory studies involving administering the drug in a controlled environment would be needed to begin to provide evidence of causation. However, in a case of this sort, the coincidence was too strong and the consequences too serious to allow the situation to continue, and the medication was withdrawn from the market.

Retrospective studies suffer from what is known as the post hoc fallacy—*post hoc, ergo propter hoc* (after this, therefore caused by this). It is extremely important for the researcher who employs this type of design to understand and remember that mere temporal sequence does not indicate causation. In the 1960s when the use of illegal drugs was for the first time being recognized as a growing phenomenon, it was commonly asserted that marijuana was a dangerous drug because use of marijuana led to heroin use and subsequent addiction. This warning was based on retrospective data from heroin addicts, who had indeed used marijuana before turning to heroin. It of course did not take into account individuals who had used marijuana and had not become heroin addicts. Further investigation into the addicts' backgrounds might have uncovered variables with an even stronger relationship to heroin addiction. It is a virtual certainty that most if not all of the addicts drank milk or attended school as children. Yet these stronger relationships were ignored in favor of a relationship that (while statistically less strong) had more intuitive appeal.

Another facet of the post hoc fallacy is the fact that so many phenomena are multiply determined. It is usually the case with human behaviors that several causes interact to produce an effect. To extend the example above in a more serious mode, it might well be true that in conjunction with some other characteristics, such as lower socioeconomic status, smoking marijuana is more likely to lead to addiction. If a researcher enters into retrospective research with a theoretical axe to grind, results may be oversimplified and an irrelevant (or at least non-causative) relationship may be given too much emphasis.

Prospective Studies

Rather than look back from the vantage point of an effect in search of a cause, as in retrospective studies, prospective studies choose a sample for whom the presumptive cause may have already occurred but for whom the effect is not yet expected to have appeared. For example, if researchers were interested in whether the incidence of the disease toxoplasmosis in pregnant women was associated with birth defects, a retrospective study would start with children exhibiting birth defects. A prospective study would begin with two groups of pregnant women—one group who had contracted the disease and another group who had not. The incidence of birth defects in the offspring of the groups would be compared. Prospective studies are methodologically stronger than retrospective studies, since the existence of a comparison group that lacks the presumptive cause (essentially an untreated control group) but appears otherwise somewhat equivalent strengthens the case for the possible causative effect of the independent variable.

Advantages and Disadvantages of Ex Post Facto Research

Both types of ex post facto study have the same design disadvantages and advantages. As previously mentioned, the mere presence of covariation between two variables does not necessarily indicate causation. Even if in fact change in one variable causes change in the other, the direction of causality is also not determinable. Often it may be found that still another unmeasured variable may have caused the variation in both measured variables.

An example of the way that the results of ex post facto research can be distorted occurred when researchers found that moderate social drinkers (of alcoholic beverages) suffered fewer heart attacks than non-drinkers. There was a strong relationship between not drinking and suffering a heart attack. The results of this study were pounced on by the popular press, who blithely announced that if you wanted to avoid a heart attack you should take up drinking!

The journalists had taken a correlation and assumed causation—that is, that drinking reduces the chances of heart attack. For these results, the converse (and equally incorrect) conclusion that heart attacks cause non-drinking, was not championed. The results probably indicate the presence of some personality factor that influences both drinking and heart attacks. One such factor might be what psychologists have labeled the Type A personality. Type A individuals are hard-driving, work-oriented, serious people. Such people are known to suffer a higher incidence of heart problems than easy-going Type B individuals. They may also be less likely to enjoy the relaxation and perceived waste of time involved in social drinking. Note that this explanation may be as incorrect or correct as any other explanation for the findings. It is offered only to illustrate how a third variable may cause variation in variables measured in an ex post facto study.

Besides the difficulties in interpreting correlational results, another disadvantage of ex post facto research is the problem of selection. Subjects assign themselves to groups through the possession of certain characteristics or behaviors. The researcher has no way of knowing all of the other characteristics the subjects also possess that might have resulted in the phenomenon of interest. In the example cited above, women who have contracted the disease toxoplasmosis are almost certainly pet owners (toxoplasmosis is contracted through contact with cat feces). Absurd as the notion might be in this case, perhaps they possess characteristics or have encountered situations other than the disease that could be related to birth defects. Or, again, drinkers may have Type B personalities or other characteristics that might be associated with a lower incidence of heart trouble. As Kerlinger (1965, p 382) so colorfully states the problem, "when assignment is not random, there is always a loophole for other variables to crawl through." Since the goal of this research is to examine the relationship between variables, this imprecision can be exasperating for the scientist.

The major advantage of ex post facto research is the possibility of a broader focus on the phenomenon than is possible with other designs. In a true experiment the researcher manipulates a variable (or several variables), hoping the variable chosen causes the variation in the dependent variable. Researchers are not always correct in their choice. Ex post facto studies can (and should) be conducted to collect data on a number of variables believed to be related to the independent variable. The calculation of the correlation coefficients will indicate which variables are, and which are not, related to the variable of interest. Thus this type of design may be more likely to yield something—even if all it can do is demonstrate covariation. Often ex post facto results are used as the basis for further studies employing more powerful true experimental or quasi-experimental designs. Moreover, in applied research it is often useful to know what factors are *not* related to your variable of interest.

□ DESCRIPTIVE RESEARCH □

Under the general heading of descriptive research fall a variety of research designs. Basically these designs have in common the fact that they seek to describe and document a phenomenon rather than specifically search for a relationship between variables. Indeed, for several types of research the entire concept of independent and dependent variables is irrelevant. The types of descriptive research to be discussed in this chapter are: (1) survey research, (2) observational research, (3) time series research, (4) secondary analysis, (5) historical research, (6) evaluation research, and (7) methodological research. For each type we will examine an overview of the research and the methods employed.

Survey Research

The term survey research has taken on a specialized meaning in recent years that actually refers to only one of the two possible forms of research conducted with the use of surveys. Status surveys are pure descriptive research in that they define the status quo. They involve polling subjects for information. A census is an example of a status survey that is designed to collect data to describe a population. Most surveys are not conducted on entire populations for very practical reasons such as time and expense. Thus most survey research is conducted on samples. Sampling procedures are therefore very important in survey research, particularly where the intent is to generalize results.

The second type of research employing surveys is that which has come to be known by the term survey research. Survey research is essentially a form of ex post facto research: it seeks to identify relationships between variables. It is discussed here because the two forms of research employing surveys employ the same methods and share the same advantages and disadvantages.

The information collected from subjects in this type of research runs the gamut from the most concrete to the most abstract. Surveys may tap demographic information, information on the subjects' environment, behaviors, level of information, attitudes, values, opinions, or motives. Even surveys focusing on one of the other forms of information usually gather at least some demographic information. This information is useful to the researcher in determining whether the sample of respondents is typical of the population. For example, if the ratio of female to male students in a nursing program is 75% to 25%, a researcher who finds that 50% of the respondents to a survey on proposed curriculum change are male would rightly question the usefulness of the data.

The methods of collecting survey information involve either direct or indirect contact with respondents. Direct methods include interviews and indirect methods include questionnaires of various types. The actual construction and content of these instruments will be discussed in Chapters 7 and 8. In this chapter we will consider more general issues.

Interviews　　Interviews can be conducted either face-to-face or via the telephone. Each method has its pros and cons. The face-to-face interview is a more intimate form of contact. It allows the interviewer to interact directly with the respondent to develop rapport. This may be particularly important if the survey items involve material about which subjects may tend to be sensitive, such as sexual issues. The trained interviewer becomes skilled at putting the respondent at ease, increasing the probability that the subjects will provide the desired information. Face-to-face contact also allows the interviewer to read the nonverbal cues of the subject that might indicate confusion or lack of understanding of the question. The interviewer may then explain or restate the question.

The major disadvantage of the face-to-face interview is the tremendous amount of effort involved on the part of the researcher. Large amounts of time are involved in contacting subjects, arranging appointments, and traveling to appointments, especially if the sample is at all large. Requiring subjects to travel to the interview may both seriously reduce the number of willing subjects and introduce selection problems, since those who are willing to go to the trouble to travel to the interview may differ from those who decline. Offering remuneration to subjects may exacerbate selection problems. The actual interview itself represents but a small fraction of the time involved with this method. Therefore data collection for studies of even moderate size may take quite a while.

The telephone interview provides the advantage of cutting down considerably on travel for the interviewer. The trade-off, however, is the loss of nonverbal cues from the respondent and a less personal contact, which may interfere with the development of rapport. Another issue is the ease with which the respondent can terminate the interview. It is much easier (not to mention more socially acceptable) to hang up a telephone than to throw someone out of your home.

The format of interviews may be either unstructured or structured. The unstructured interview is more of an informal chat in which, although certain types of information are sought, the order in which questions are asked is not fixed and the tolerance for irrelevant information is high. This is not to say that unstructured interviews are always informal in tone. Often employment interviews are unstructured. Perhaps a better term would be flexible. Subjects and interviewers are freer to explore some topics in more depth than others and to add topics.

The structured interview is much less flexible. The order of questions is fixed, as is the format of the questions. Such measures ensure standard information from all subjects but may result in a much more stilted, formal interview. Skillful arrangement of questions on sensitive topics may increase the probability that subjects will cooperate. The art of interview design will be discussed in Chapter 7.

The interviewer must be trained before data collection begins. The interviewer must be familiar with the subject matter in order to be sure all necessary data is collected. In addition the interviewer must exhibit the proper demeanor during the interview to ensure that data gathered are of acceptable quality. The interviewer must not be intimidating to the subject, particularly in the case of sensitive questions. The interviewer must be friendly enough to establish rapport, yet formal enough to impress the subject with the importance of the session. The interviewer must be trained to read the nonverbal cues of the subject but must learn not to provide cues to the subject (such as disapproval) that might cause the subject to alter responses to please the interviewer. The interviewer must practice enough with the instrument so as to provide standardized treatment to subjects to help minimize instrumentation effects. Practice with peers or with videotape equipment is often extremely helpful.

The major disadvantage of the interview is similar to that of questionnaire data. Whenever asking subjects to self-report, the researcher must worry about the honesty of the responses. This is more of a problem for some topics than others. An interviewer from the IRS who is asking a respondent whether he has cheated on his taxes can expect less candor than an interviewer asking a randomly selected city dweller her opinion on the new statue erected in front of city hall. Honesty is not the only problem, however. There are a number of response biases, as will be discussed in Chapter 9. Some subjects will agree with anything, some will agree with nothing, and some will not venture an opinion or provide information on any topic.

Questionnaires   Questionnaires may at first glance appear to be nothing more than self-administered interviews. Actually, there is a great deal of difference between the methods—and some of these differences might well mandate the use of one instrument over another.

Questionnaires are less sensitive instruments than interviews. They are essentially impersonal, so the rapport that may be established by the interviewer is lost. The forms, since subjects self-administer them, must be clear and understandable. Subjects will at times feel they "lose face" by admitting they do not understand a questionnaire and will attempt to complete it anyway. This sensitivity is even more pronounced when the subject has trouble reading the questionnaire. There is an appalling lack of literacy in the general population. Many people simply cannot read or do so at such a level as to render filling out a questionnaire a herculean task. That questionnaires are written by overeducated researchers unaware that a problem exists often makes the problem worse. A disadvantage of questionnaires is that, when reading a completed form, the researcher may have no idea that the responses were based on misunderstood instructions or questions. Pilot testing of researcher-developed questionnaires on several individuals characteristic of the population of interest is vital for this reason. Questionnaire design will be discussed in Chapter 8.

Classically, questionnaires have been distributed by mail with a stamped return envelope addressed to the researcher to facilitate returns. The return rate for questionnaire studies is always a matter of concern. Return rates of between 20% and 35% are not uncommon. Thus although the questionnaire is less time intensive for the researcher than interviews, it may be quite costly to duplicate and distribute (with postage) forms that may well never be seen again. A further problem associated with a low return rate is the question of who returns the forms. The researcher must check to assure that the sample is typical of the population on important characteristics.

More recently, researchers have attempted to increase returns and introduce some level of personal contact through delivering forms to respondents and picking up (or waiting for) completed forms. This procedure introduces all the costs associated with interviews without gaining the advantages of the interview.

The major vehicle at the researcher's disposal to encourage participation by subjects is the cover letter. This should be addressed as personally as possible (not "Dear Sir or Madam") and should explain the research and emphasize the importance of cooperation. (A useful, albeit somewhat manipulative, ploy to increase cooperation is to convince respondents they are doing you a great service with their cooperation and earning your undying gratitude. In other words, grovel.) As mentioned above, always include a stamped return envelope.

Survey Issues   Sampling is an issue for both interviews and questionnaire surveys. Anything that the researcher can do to facilitate the use of probability sampling techniques (Chapter 3) will strengthen the design. A check should be run on the returned questionnaires and on completed interviews to determine whether the sample sufficiently resembles the population of interest.

An important issue in survey-type research involves the subjects' anonymity and the confidentiality of information provided by subjects. This is a very serious ethical issue. As will be discussed further in Chapter 10, subjects must be assured that information they provide will be available only to the research staff. They should be assured that their identity will not be recognizable in any published account of the research. Not only are such assurances ethically mandated, but they also tend to have the immensely practical effect of relaxing subjects and increasing candor.

Observational Methods

Observational methods differ from survey-based research in that observational methods do not rely on subjects' self-reports. This tends to render them somewhat less biased than surveys. However, let us hasten to add, the observer can serve as a source of bias, as will be discussed in Chapter 9.

Several techniques can be used to minimize the amount of subjectivity introduced by the observer. Rather than being asked to describe behaviors labeled by such subjective terms as "dependent" or "depressed," the observer should be supplied with an instrument that lists concrete behaviors to be either checked off at occurrence or rated on a frequency scale. This prevents the observer from employing some subjective, idiosyncratic definition of the construct.

Before the observer is allowed to rate actual subjects, rigorous training should be provided. Often video tapes are useful for this purpose. The observer rates the tapes, and the ratings are checked by the researcher. It is important both that the observer rate reliably and that the observer be correct. The use of many observers who have been trained to a level of reliability with each other reduces subjectivity in ratings, as does the use of several sessions in rating a particular subject.

Repeated sessions with the subject are useful for another reason. Being watched can be a very unsettling experience; until the subjects become accustomed to the presence of an observer, their behaviors may be atypical.

Case Study or Report   A special example of a type of research that uses observational techniques (in conjunction with other techniques) is the case study or report. In this research an individual patient or institution or setting is examined in detail. Case studies often concern unusual or unique occurrences or situations. For this reason the results of the study are not readily generalizable. However, the very uniqueness of the subject often reduces the importance of this fact. Case studies may be used as the starting point for further research, having called attention to the condition or situation.

The document resulting from a case study is fairly standardized as to format, regardless of the subject matter (although the terminology may appear to imply application only to patients). The report contains historical data about the subject as well as present demographic data. The situation or individual's diagnosis is noted, along with any measures or tests administered. The treatment approach is laid out with notes on treatment administration. Finally a statement of the conclusion of the case or a prognosis is given. The case study is frequently encountered in the health sciences literature.

Time Series Research

As was mentioned in Chapter 5, uninterrupted time series data are primarily employed in forecasting. Time series data consist of repeated measurements of a phenomenon over a period of time. For example, in justifying a request for more staff, the chief of a physical therapy department might demonstrate that over the last two years, the number of patients served by the staff has shown a steady increase of 10% per month. On the basis of these data it might be reasonable to forecast a continued increase in usage and therefore a need for additional staff. Forecasting methods based on time series are also employed to determine how much food to buy for the hospital cafeteria for the next week, and how much annual income the hospital forecasts for the next year as the basis for departmental allocations.

Secondary Analysis

In secondary analysis the researcher does not collect data. Data collected previously by others is reanalyzed. When conducting a study researchers often collect more data than they can handle, and they may only analyze or report on some subset of the whole. Secondary analysis may examine data using different hypotheses, a different subset of subjects, different statistical techniques, or a change in the unit of analysis. Secondary analysis is being facilitated by the establishment of data libraries such as the International Data Library and Reference Service at the University of California at Berkeley or the Council of Social Science Data Archives in New York City. Often, however, researchers are willing to provide their raw data to individuals wishing to do a secondary analysis upon request.

Clearly, this is a less expensive form of research, since it involves no collection of data. However, by not collecting data the researcher relinquishes control and often wishes the original researcher had collected data on just one more variable, or had collected the data in a slightly different form.

Historical Research

Historical research is "undertaken in order to test hypotheses or to answer questions concerning causes, effects, or trends relating to past events that may shed light on present behaviors or practices" (Polit & Hungler 1983, p 202). Often understanding of present behaviors or attitudes can be increased through an examination of the past. For example, the present-day resistance on the part of neighborhoods to allowing the establishment of half-way houses for psychiatric patients may be based on the past use of the medical model, which referred to "mental illness." Or it may have its basis even further in the past, in a time when psychiatric disturbances were viewed as demonic possession. In either case present attitudes may be based on some fear of contamination through contact.

Historical research is based on primary and secondary sources. Primary sources are documents, remains or relics, and oral testimony. Primary sources must be first-hand accounts such as autobiographies or affidavits. Secondary sources are documents about the subject not based on direct experience.

Sources are evaluated through the use of external and internal criticism. External criticism is based on determining the validity or authenticity of the source. Was it actually written by a witness? Could the document have been forged?

Internal criticism establishes the truth of the authentic document. Is there any reason this person might lie? Could this person actually have known this information? To establish its truth, the document is compared to other accounts of the era and of the phenomenon of interest. It is not uncommon for sources to contradict each other. When this occurs, the decision on which to believe is a matter for the researcher's best judgment.

A major problem with historical research is sampling. In this context sampling refers to the sources. It is wise to employ as many primary sources as is practical. This may not be as easy as it sounds, however. Documents get lost or destroyed. People die. A dearth of sources can hinder the credibility of the research.

Evaluation Research

Evaluation research asks one of two questions—"What should we do?" or "How are we doing?" The first question refers to what is known as formative evaluation research. This represents the collection of data or opinion to be used to determine a policy or to design a program. Service providers as well as recipients are given a forum (or should be) to present their ideas.

A subtype of formative evaluation research is known as need assessment. As the name implies, this type of research involves determining what resources are required. This information can be gathered from a few involved individuals (known as key informants) or through the use of surveys.

The question of "how we're doing" is assessed through summative evaluation research, which involves evaluating an existing program or policy. The traditional approach to summative evaluation research involves a four-step process. The first step involves determining the goals of the policy or program and stating them in such a way that they may be used as criteria for accomplishments. This involves writing the goals in the form known as behavioral objectives. These are the same thing as operational definitions. Goals must be more concrete than "making patients happier" or you can never determine when the goal has been accomplished. Often this first step is surprisingly difficult. There appears to be some relation between the ability to state goals and the ability to accomplish them. Once goals are stated, measures can be designed or obtained that assess the degree to which the goals have been attained. These measures are employed to collect data, which are analyzed and compared to the goals.

An invasion of outside evaluators into a program is often very threatening to those involved in the program. Defensiveness on the part of program personnel can make summative evaluation research difficult to carry out.

Then there is the problem of what to do with the results. Fortunately, this is not usually the researcher's problem. The role of the researcher is to provide results; it is the job of the policy-maker to utilize them. How far below the full attainment of goals should a program be allowed to fall before funding is cut, thereby removing services and eliminating jobs? If a program has several stated goals and fully meets one but falls short on others, what then? What if the goals of the program can't be delineated? These are policy questions, not research questions.

Methodological Research

Methodological research develops, validates, and evaluates standardized measures. Such research establishes the validity and reliability of research instruments, which improves the quality of research in the discipline by reducing instrumentation threats and allowing researchers access to instruments that allow comparability across studies and eliminate the need to employ questionable home-grown instruments. In addition, methodological research works on the scaling of instruments and sharpens their construct validity. Methodological research is particularly important in disciplines, such as the health sciences, that are just evolving into "scientific" disciplines and beginning to perform research. Although methodological research will not be discussed in detail in this text, it is important to recognize that it may be one of the most significant contributors to the evolution of health science research as an exact science.

□ SUMMARY □

Non-experimental research involves measurement or observation of variables rather than manipulation of variables by the investigator. For this reason causative explanations for results are not appropriate.

The two major categories of non-experimental research are ex post facto research in which relationships between variables are sought, and descriptive research. The two subtypes of ex post facto research, prospective and retrospective, share the problem of the post hoc fallacy. Since any relationship between variables is correlational in nature, the tendency to assume causation must be avoided.

Descriptive research includes (1) survey research, which employs interviews and questionnaires to collect data; (2) observational research; (3) time series research, which measures a phenomenon or process over a period of time; (4) secondary analysis, in which data gathered by others are re-analyzed and interpreted; (5) historical research; (6) evaluation research, which gauges the progress and effectiveness of programs and interventions such as legislation; and (7) methodological research, which seeks to strengthen the scientific foundations of the research instrumentation and procedures within various disciplines.

□ KEY TERMS □

ex post facto research	observational research
descriptive research	case study or report
retrospective studies	time series research
post hoc fallacy	secondary analysis
prospective studies	historical research
survey research	evaluation research
status surveys	formative evaluation research
interviews	summative evaluation research
questionnaires	methodological research

□□ 7 □□
Interviews

The interview is an extremely useful tool in collecting research data. As mentioned in Chapter 6, it can yield information that could not be collected by any other means. As the interaction between two individuals, interviews involve special nuances in the process of collecting data. In this chapter we will focus on the individuals involved in the process, methods of structuring the content of the interview to maximize the effectiveness of data collection, and interviewer techniques that facilitate the process. Interviews and written questionnaires and tests share a number of characteristics. Those forms and procedures that apply most frequently to interviews will be covered in this chapter; techniques that apply more commonly to written instruments will be covered in Chapter 8. Because of the overlap and occasionally somewhat arbitrary decisions on where information could best be presented, Chapters 7 and 8 should be viewed as a functional unit.

□ INTERVIEW PARTICIPANTS □

The effectiveness of the interview in eliciting the information desired by the researcher depends on both the interviewer and the respondent. As human beings, both participants have any number of demographic and personality characteristics that may affect their behavior during the interview. The unique interaction of these characteristics will undoubtedly result in data that will differ from those that would result from any other pairing of the same interviewer or respondent with other individuals. Such variability may to some extent be controlled through the design and structure of the interview itself.

Interviewers

Given the recognition of the importance of a good interviewer to the quality of the data collected, it is surprising how little agreement exists about the characteristics that describe the ideal interviewer. This is partly due to the differences in types of interviews (e.g., employment interviews vs. counseling interviews) and topics that have been employed in the research process. The skills needed to conduct a market research interview may differ significantly from those that will be called into play during an interview of parents designed to assess the impairment of a handicapped child. We shall first examine those interviewer characteristics that have been systematically examined through research, then develop a job description enumerating the skills generally needed by the interviewer.

At the outset of the interview respondents know little about the interviewer other than the role definition and any characteristics that they may infer from the interviewer's appearance. Although interviewers generally possess somewhat more information about the respondent, they, too, may respond to immediately visible characteristics. In other words, both participants may rely on visual cues as the basis for attributing personality characteristics to the other. The most obvious such characteristics are race, gender, and age.

Race of interviewer has been shown to interact with respondent characteristics to affect interview data. The effect has been found to be strongest on racially related topics. Blacks tend to respond more militantly to black interviewers than to white interviewers (Hagenaars & Hanen, 1982). White respondents of higher educational levels will tend to give more liberal responses to black than to white interviewers. Such effects would need to be considered in the design of the study and the selection of interviewers. In interviews of aged white respondents, for example, it was found that black interviewers experienced difficulty in eliciting responses (Hagenaars & Hanen, 1982).

Gender of interviewer has shown few consistent effects on the interview process. Observed effects have depended on the interview topic. On interviews about sexuality, it was found that male interviewers were able to elicit fewer responses from female respondents than were female interviewers.

Age of interviewer is strongly associated with experience and skill—that is, younger interviewers may not possess the skills of older interviewers, and less skilled interviewers are more likely to quit. Here, too, however, when effects have been observed, better data appear to be obtained when there is some matching of interviewer and respondent. In interviews of teenage girls, Ehrlich and Reisman (1961) found that younger interviewers obtained more peer-oriented responses than did older interviewers.

Three less immediately obvious characteristics that have been investigated are the interviewer's personality characteristics, attitudes, and expectations. The personality factors that have consistently been shown to affect interview quality are intelligence and self-confidence. Both of these characteristics are associated with obtaining more data in terms of both amount and quality of data. The interviewer's attitudes have been found to be related to demand characteristics (see Chapter 9). Strong attitudes on the part of the interviewer often elicit matching attitudes from respondents. For this reason the well-trained interviewer will have learned to present a neutral position so as to elicit the respondent's true position.

Interviewers' expectations about the interview are also often confirmed by cooperative subjects. Interviewers who expect refusals, reluctance to respond to certain material or unwillingness to participate in general find these behaviors occurring significantly more frequently than do interviewers who do not.

Since identifying characteristics of interviewers appears not to provide much information about the "best" interviewer, another approach is to identify the skills necessary to conduct an effective interview and seek those skills in potential interviewers. Richardson, Dohrenwend, and Klein (1965) have developed a list of eight skills required of the interviewer. These requirements are a mix of personality traits and skills acquired through training.

The skills are (1) knowledge of the subject matter, (2) conceptual and analytical ability, (3) ability to translate concepts into content areas and questions, (4) ability to gain and exploit new ideas and insights during the interview, (5) skill in formulating questions during the interview, (6) skill in selecting respondents, (7) ability to gain the participation of respondents, and (8) skill in recording data from the interview. The extent to which any one of these skills is important depends on the structure and rigidity of the format of the interview and the role of the interviewer vis a vis the researcher. Various forms of interview are discussed later in this chapter.

Respondents

Investigators into the effects of respondent characteristics have focused on the extent to which these characteristics tend to result in the response biases discussed later in this chapter. Again, race has been found to interact with interviewer's race. Black respondents have been found to show less acquiescence bias (tendency to agree) when interviewed by black interviewers (Carr, 1971). Generally, gender of respondent does not appear to result in differences in respondent behavior, except on threatening material, where women are more likely than men to provide the socially desirable response. All subjects are more likely to acquiesce when items are worded positively.

In research specifically examining sociomedical items (Hochstim & Renne, 1971), no differences based on the respondents' gender were found. There was an effect for respondent level of education, however, with less well educated respondents proving less reliable in their responses.

In summary, it appears that the skills of the interviewer probably outweigh other factors in obtaining good data. In cases of sensitive or threatening topics, however, the evidence at least suggests that some sort of matching of demographic characteristics of interviewer and respondent may result in more valid data.

▪ INTERVIEW STRUCTURE ▪

Richardson, Dohrenwend, and Klein (1965) have described two categories of interview: unstandardized and standardized. The unstandardized interview does not necessarily seek to obtain the same information from every respondent. It may be employed to define the parameters of a phenomenon that will later serve as the focus for a more standardized interview. In other words, the researcher who becomes prematurely committed to a particular focus or investigative framework before gaining a clear idea of the possible components of a phenomenon might well miss some important facets of the situation. For example, an investigator concerned with community perceptions of the adequacy of health care in a community might well begin with unstructured interviews that allow respondents to air their areas of concern. Once these concerns are delineated, later interviews might ask respondents to deal with these areas in particular. Because the unstandardized interview is complex and somewhat amorphous, a clear set of routine practices cannot really be developed.

The standardized interview is designed to collect the same information from each respondent on a specific set of issues in such a form that results are comparable and classifiable. The structured interview is thus a more useful research instrument. The procedures for the design of structured interviews have been clearly established.

There are two forms of standardized interview. Although both collect the same information, the process and formats differ. The nonschedule standardized interview does not follow a precise and invariant format. The interviewer is extensively trained about the material that must be collected, but is then free to determine the order and the wording of questions. In the schedule standardized interview the wording for each question and the precise order in which questions will be presented are predetermined.

One reason for the adoption of the schedule standardized interview involves the standardization of interviewer behavior. To the extent that interviewers vary even such subtle signifiers as facial expression and voice tone, irrelevant (and possibly systematic) noise enters the data. If a respondent does not hear or understand a question in a schedule standardized interview (in its purest form) the experimenter/interviewer may only reread the question as it appears on the schedule. In research design terms, the treatment is kept identical (or as much so as possible given uncontrollable individual interviewer differences) for all respondents.

The use of the schedule standardized interview is based on four assumptions (Richardson et al, 1965). The first is that respondents in a study will be sufficiently homogeneous that it will be possible to formulate questions in a way that respondents will understand. It is essential to pretest questions on a representative sample of respondents in a manner that will allow the interviewer to ascertain what the respondents perceived to be the meaning of the question. Misinterpretations—either systematic or random—will distort the data. The issue of question wording is dealt with later in this chapter.

The second assumption (resting on the first) is that the respondents' vocabulary can be constructed into a question that will "work" for all respondents. Just because respondents all recognize the terminology of a question does not mean that they will all interpret it in the same way. Extreme formality or informality in the phrasing of a question may confuse or offend some respondents.

The third assumption is based on the ordering of questions. If the meaning of a question is to be identical for all respondents, the context must be identical. Thus the order must be invariant between respondents. The final assumption is that it is possible (through pilot testing) to meet the first three assumptions. (Pilot testing refers to pretesting components of the research in advance of formal data collection.)

Whether it is possible to meet the assumptions of the schedule standardized interview is a matter of controversy. It can be argued that if the goal is to have the respondent understand the question, it must be worded in a manner familiar to the respondent. The issue is whether through standardization of wording one can standardize meaning. In the case where a respondent clearly indicates lack of understanding, the interviewer employing a schedule standardized interview has no alternative but to reread the question. With a nonschedule standardized interview the interviewer is free to rephrase the question so that the respondent understands it.

In discussing the ordering of questions, proponents of the nonschedule approach would argue that there is no perfect format for all respondents. The skilled interviewer can ascertain from the respondent willingness to pursue a particular line of questioning and should be free to reorder questions to maximize respondent cooperation.

Recall that both the schedule and nonschedule standardized interviews collect data on the same set of questions. What, then, determines which format to adopt? The major difference between the formats pertains to the point in the process where the most expertise is required. In the schedule format, by the time the interviewer is faced with a respondent, all relevant decisions have been made. The procedure is so completely standardized that less initiative and flexibility is required of the interviewer. Training of interviewers takes less time, and less highly trained interviewers command lower rates of pay. The interviewer using the nonschedule format must possess a far higher level of experience and expertise in order to determine the most effective wording and format for each respondent. Thus the nonschedule format becomes more expensive to administer. Unfortunately, it is often this difference in cost that determines the choice of format rather than more directly research-related concerns. If the best possible data are to be collected, the choice should be governed by the extent of homogeneity of respondents and the topic of the interview.

Interview Questions

There are two basic types of questions that may be used in interviews—the open-ended and the closed question. Open-ended questions allow respondents to formulate their answers in whatever way they choose. With closed questions, respondents are presented with a selection of alternative responses and invited to choose one. In this chapter we will focus on open-ended questions. Because the use of closed questions is much more common in written data collection instruments, the formatting of these questions will be described in Chapter 8.

Open-ended questions are useful in many contexts, alone and in conjunction with closed questions. Stanley Payne, in *The Art of Asking Questions*, lists a number of varieties of open-ended questions: (1) introductory questions, (2) suggestions or recommendations for action on a specific topic, (3) elaboration on preceding questions, (4) explanations for previous responses, (5) argument questions, (6) knowledge questions, (7) sources of respondents' information, and (8) factual information. Open-ended questions are particularly useful (and important) for dealing with complex information where nuances might be lost by forcing respondents to choose among predefined response categories.

Labaw (1980) cites three important uses of open-ended questions: (1) to explore complex issues, (2) to measure intensity of respondent feeling, and (3) to identify lack of understanding. Some questions that appear to deal with a single issue actually represent a complex of interrelated concerns. Labaw cites as an example the seemingly straightforward question, "What are your feelings toward abortion?" As she points out, however, the issue of abortion touches on such concerns as "killing and murder, issues of mental and physical health, and issues of world overpopulation and limited food supply" (p 130). Even if the interviewer has included a multitude of closed questions touching the potentially relevant areas, the open question identifies the areas of concern for the individual respondent.

Open-ended questions not only measure the intensity of emotion surrounding an issue but may be the only way to tap respondent ambivalence. If the respondent must choose a response category, he or she will likely choose (at least momentarily) the stronger or more salient of a complex of emotions.

Lack of understanding or unclear definition of terms on the part of respondents can be identified in several ways through the use of open questions. If the respondent's answer appears to be unrelated to the question, it may be that he or she has misunderstood the question. Even more directly, the respondent may simply admit to not understanding a question or term. Such candor is less common in the more structured questionnaire setting.

Coding Open-Ended Responses

Responses to open-ended questions must be converted into a data form suitable for analysis. This is done through the process of coding, a dull, tedious task that is also vitally important. Poor or insensitive coding may totally undermine the time and care taken to collect the uncoded data.

The poorest form of coding is called word coding. It involves looking through the responses until certain key words indicate to the coder a category into which the data are coded. Much more useful, and difficult, is concept coding. This involves looking past the wording of the response to the underlying concepts. Concept coding may actually provide for fewer response categories than word coding but it certainly provides more meaningful codes. Concept coding requires much more training and expertise than does word coding, but the researcher concerned with high-quality data should seriously consider the expenditure of necessary resources (training for coders or using the researcher's own time for coding).

Wording of Questions

The actual wording of interview questions may be a major determining factor in the collection of appropriate data. Because researchers generally are well educated, and often somewhat isolated, the language employed in interviews and questionnaires is often a barrier to subject response. As Richardson points out, "language usage varies with geographic region, social background, special interests and occupations and level of education" (p 224). Each of these differences may require a translation of the interview question into the local vernacular. Four areas of language usage should be monitored carefully by the investigator.

The use of slang or street language may or may not be appropriate, depending on the characteristics of the interview's respondents. Including slang terms may decrease the level of formality of the interview yet at the same time increase respondent understanding and rapport. Interviewers, however, should not attempt to employ language with which they are not entirely comfortable. Awkwardness may be interpreted by respondents as scorn and might create resentment, and the unidiomatic use of slang can create a sense of alienation exactly opposite to the effect being sought.

The deliberate use of less formal terms may, in some cases, be a necessity. Mothers being interviewed about toilet training might find the phrase "elimination of feces" totally incomprehensible but respond to a less formal term such as "bowel movement".

Professionals employ a lot of jargon—words assigned an idiosyncratic definition known only to the select few. The use of jargon should be avoided. Even when used with other professional groups, jargon appears to be exactly what it is—an exclusionary device whose usage is discriminatory. When actual status differences already exist, use of jargon may be even more inflammatory. Acronyms should also be avoided unless the title for which the acronym stands is paired with it on the first several presentations.

Finally, the use of highly emotionally charged words should be avoided. A fine example of this error is presented by Koller (1960) in a study of the parents of children with physical disabilities that was designed to assess the parents' expectations of a rehabilitation center service. The study sent out letters requesting participation and met with a very high refusal rate. Finally one parent admitted to refusing because the letterhead employed the word "cripple" and she could not think of her child in those terms. The letterhead was changed and the refusal rate dropped dramatically.

Sequencing the Interview

The order in which questions are presented in an interview is extremely important. The goal of the interview is to collect information from the subject. Thus the questions should draw the respondent into the process and reduce the probability of premature termination of the interview. As the subject moves through the interview, early questions may affect the respondent's reactions to later questions. Thus the interviewer must be alert for any potential biasing effect of questions. Clearly these issues are most formally salient for the schedule standardized interview. However, they are also important for the interviewer in the nonschedule format who wishes to retain the respondent and collect unbiased data.

Generally the first several questions are designed to elicit the interest of the subject in continuing the interview. They should be broad, general questions that do not require a great deal of thought or inspire strong feelings. The goal is to involve the subject and to establish rapport. (This order may *not* be appropriate when the topic is so emotion laden that subjects must be given the opportunity to express themselves before they can concentrate on the interview.) These initial questions need not be thought of as dispensable. The information obtained may provide a baseline to determine whether topics brought out in the interview in any way altered the respondents' initial response.

Threatening or sensitive questions or topics should generally be introduced after rapport has been established and the respondent appears comfortable. For threatening topics, open-ended questions have been shown to elicit more accurate data as they reduce the effect of a social desirability bias (to be discussed in Chapter 8). However, respondents are also more likely to refuse to answer when the questions are on a sensitive topic. For threatening topics it has also been shown that increasing the question length increases respondents' willingness to respond (Bradburn & Sudman, 1979).

The above-mentioned techniques represent what Labaw (1980) refers to as routing to avoid refusals and terminations. Another use of routing is to break up mind sets that the respondents might establish. Often it is necessary in an interview to ask the respondent to respond to lists of items in terms of ratings. The respondent may very quickly begin to respond automatically without thinking about each alternative. Such mind sets can be broken by routing the respondent through the interview so that such lists are interspersed with other material that requires different types of response. Also, statements can be ordered so that negative and positive statements are distributed within the list in such a way that the respondent must consider each item separately.

Finally, routing may be used to avoid the sequencing effect mentioned above. If an interview was intended to determine attitudes toward health care facilities, a poor interview would begin by asking about high health-care costs and hospital understaffing and then ask the respondent to discuss problems in the health care system.

It is inevitable that as the respondent moves through the interview, a process of education takes place. The interviewer runs the risk of affecting attitudes or even creating attitudes that did not previously exist. This problem can be somewhat reduced through question ordering. The effect can be measured by beginning and ending the interview with a general question and comparing responses to see if the interview itself has affected earlier attitudes or beliefs.

Five types of sequencing effects have been identified. The evidence for each as summarized by Molenaar (1982) appears inconclusive, but there is a sufficient number of examples of each to suggest that when a series of questions deals with related subject matter, such effects can, in fact, occur. These effects are: (1) the saliency effect, (2) the reference group effect, (3) the consistency effect, (4) the contrast effect, and (5) the rapport effect.

The saliency effect involves early questions that focus the respondent's attention on specific aspects of subsequent questions, perhaps by encouraging the creation of a particular mental set on the part of the respondent. An example would be to ask about major problems in the respondent's life and then ask questions about the respondent's job or relationships. A saliency effect would incline the respondent to respond to the later questions with the preconception of a "problem," and should thus result in more negative responses.

The reference group effect refers to the norms of a reference group made salient by previous questions. For example, DeLamater (1974) found that women espoused a more conservative sexual ideology when previous questions had dealt with the ideology of their best friends. This effect can work in both directions depending on how the respondent feels toward the reference group invoked. If a disliked reference group is invoked, respondents may move their position away from the perceived position of the reference group.

Consistency effects involve pointing out the relationship between two related cognitions (thoughts) or attitudes in sequenced questions. According to cognitive dissonance theory (Festinger, 1959), individuals become uncomfortable when faced with inconsistencies in their attitudes or cognitions. To reduce this discomfort, one of the cognitions (or attitudes) is altered and brought into line with the other cognition so that the source of the dissonance is removed.

The contrast effect results when an early question highlights the contrast between the meaning or subject of earlier and later questions.

In the final effect, the rapport effect, the earlier questions may increase rapport between the interviewer and respondent such that later responses may be more candid.

□ THE INTERVIEW PROCESS □

Up to this point we have been primarily concerned with the identity of the interview participants and the content of the interview. It is also important to consider aspects of the interaction itself—the process of the interview.

There are two components of the pacing of the interview. The first is the general tempo or speed of the actual question and answer process, the second is the speed with which topic changes or transitions are accomplished. In terms of general tempo, interviewers are likely to err in the direction of too quick a tempo. Interviewers are generally well-educated, intelligent individuals who are well trained and quite familiar with the interview content. The respondent will often lack these advantages—particularly familiarity with content. Thus the respondent may need to move more slowly than the interviewer recognizes. This may result in the respondent feeling rushed and unimportant. Excessive speed in conducting the interview may result in the respondent's becoming confused, insecure, or angry, depending on how he or she interprets the reasons for the speed. Any of these responses may result in distorted data. The sensitive interviewer must watch for cues from the respondent as to comfort with the pace. Usually the final pacing represents a compromise between the preferred pacing of the interviewer and that of the respondent.

Transitions or changes in topic are generally introduced by the interviewer. Such changes must be made skillfully. The respondent should feel that the current topic has been exhausted, or else he or she may feel that the interviewer is not paying attention. If the respondent feels cut off, further participation may be seriously reduced.

Transitions should be logical and smooth, and topics should be logically related — abrupt transitions may jar the respondent and reduce participation. In cases where a topic appears to be causing the respondent severe anxiety, however, an abrupt transition to a safer topic is appropriate.

Occasionally the respondent will introduce a change in topic. In schedule formats the respondent must be returned to the previous position in the schedule. In nonschedule formats it is important for the interviewer to determine the reason for the change. Respondents may switch topics because they feel they've exhausted the present topic, because they are bored, or because they find another topic more interesting. In these cases it is appropriate to allow the transition. It is also possible for respondents to employ transitions to escape threatening material. If this is the case, the interviewer may wish to return to the topic later in the interview when the respondent is more comfortable.

In addition to the questions themselves, interviewers employ other verbal techniques to control the respondent's behavior in the interview. Interviewers may reinforce or lengthen participation through encouragements and silences, and discourage participation through the use of "guggles" (Richardson et al, 1965) and interruptions.

Encouragements are words or phrases intended to reinforce the respondents' participation. Comments such as "I see" or "Good" may convey interest, comprehension, and encouragement for the respondent to continue. Such encouragements tend to lengthen respondents' replies.

Encouragements appear most useful when the initial interaction between the interviewer and respondent is neutral in nature and the respondent is somewhat reluctant to participate. When the initial interaction is positive and the respondent is quite talkative, encouragements are unnecessary. In the unfortunate situation where the initial interaction between interviewer and respondent has a negative tone, verbal encouragements are ineffective in increasing participation.

The use of silence to increase subject participation is a delicate business. Short silences (about 3 seconds) that are broken by the respondent do tend to lengthen responses. Longer silences tend to be broken by the interviewer. Regardless of who breaks the silence, however, these longer silences actually serve to shorten responses.

"Guggle" is a term borrowed by Richardson and associates (1965) from Gilbert and Sullivan to describe short sounds (such as "ah") that the interviewer employs to indicate a desire to speak. Guggles do not represent actual interruptions of the respondent's speech but rather serve as cues to shorten the response. Interruptions, of course, involve actually breaking into the respondent's reply.

If guggles and interruptions are employed sparingly and for purposes of clarifying responses, they generally do not serve to reduce respondent participation. Frequent use, however, will tend to inhibit respondents.

The goal of the interview is to collect the desired data. Two types of respondents present difficulties in this regard: garrulous and reticent respondents. Respondents of the first type talk too much, those of the second, too little. The techniques just described may be employed to assist in data collection with these individuals.

A respondent may talk too much for several reasons. If he or she is lonely or isolated, the interview may represent a rare opportunity for human interaction. In such a case (if time permits) a conversation before beginning the interview may reduce some of the need to talk. Garrulity may also represent an attempt by the respondent to create a diversion.

Silences will not work with the over-talkative respondent, who will simply continue to talk. Guggles should be employed, and when the respondent pauses for breath, the interviewer should break in to summarize the response and immediately pose another question. Another technique is to increase the use of closed questions.

The concern with the reticent respondent is to draw the person out. The silent respondent may be naturally quiet, may be participating in the interview under duress of some kind, or may be threatened by the interview topic. The interviewer should seek to initiate interactions through the use of closed questions. As the respondent loosens up, the interviewer can offer encouragements and can switch to open-ended questions. With either type of client the use of a schedule standardized format is extremely difficult (if not impossible).

Interviews represent an important method of data collection. In Chapter 8 we turn to a discussion of data collection through written instruments and hardware (equipment). Closed questions, which may be employed in either interviews or questionnaires, and written instruments will be discussed at length.

□ SUMMARY □

Interviews can be an extremely effective data collection device. Because they entail direct interaction between two people, they provide a unique means of collecting otherwise unavailable data. Characteristics of the interviewer and the respondent interact to enhance or damage the effectiveness of this tool.

Interviews may be either unstandardized or standardized. In the unstandardized format, the data collected from various subjects may involve different topics and issues and therefore be uncomparable across subjects. Standardized interviews collect uniform information from respondents and therefore represent a superior research tool. The actual format, wording of questions, and order of questions is invariant in the schedule standardized interview. In the nonschedule standardized interview, the interviewers are free to employ their expertise in determining order and wording of questions to enhance respondents' cooperation and comprehension.

□ KEY TERMS □

unstandardized interview	sequence effect
standardized interview	saliency effect
schedule standardized interview	reference group effect
nonschedule standardized	consistency effect
interview	contrast effect
open-ended questions	rapport effect
concept coding	"guggles"
word coding	
routing	

□□ 8 □□
Hardware and Written Data Collection Instruments

□ *Hardware Instrumentation*
□ *Written Instruments*
□ *Test Validity*
□ *Locating Written Instruments*
□ *Developing Written Instruments*
  □ *Question Format*
  □ *Item Wording*
  □ *Response Formats*
□ *Evaluating Instruments*
□ *Response Bias*

In health-sciences research, two important sources of data are physical measures and written instruments such as surveys, inventories, and standardized tests. In this chapter we will discuss the decisions and issues involved in selecting hardware instrumentation for the collection of physical measures, in locating and evaluating written instruments, and in developing specialized written instrumentation.

□ HARDWARE INSTRUMENTATION □

Many research studies in the health sciences employ physical measures of such functions as joint motion or lung capacity as their dependent measures. In many of the ways previously discussed such "hard" measures are preferable to self-report variables because they are less vulnerable to sub-

112

jects' biases. Physical measures are also desirable because of the relative ease with which the measures can be operationally defined.

In defining physical measures, the physical, mechanical instrument involved in the actual measurement process represents an extremely important component of the research. Because of technological advancement in medical science, there are many such instruments that may be employed in research, such as cable tensiometers, spirometers, electroencephalographs (EEGs), and goniometers.

When a dependent variable is being defined in terms of a physical process there is theoretically a choice between using already developed equipment and designing and constructing custom equipment. For most investigators, the latter is not really a viable option for a number of reasons. The technological expertise required in electronics and design may well be beyond the capabilities of the investigator, and resources for assistance may be unavailable. Even when such knowledge and skill are available, however, the time required to design and perfect instrumentation may be prohibitive (unless the goal of the research is methodological advancement). The costs involved may also be a realistic cause for concern.

Given that the researcher generally will employ previously developed devices and equipment, where does he or she obtain information on the options available? The purchasing department of institutions that employ equipment (hospitals and universities) have copies of the catalogs published by manufacturers of various types of equipment. The firms employ representatives who may be quite helpful in defining and fulfilling equipment needs. Authors of articles in the various journals will usually be more than willing to supply information on equipment they have employed in published studies if such information is unavailable in the research report.

Finally, there are several resources available to investigators that list equipment available along with the manufacturers' names and addresses. Reilly Publications Co., (Park Ridge, IL 60068) publishes a semi-monthly paper, *Medical Electronics and Equipment News*, which is available by subscription. The paper reports on the availability of instruments including scientific apparatus, electronic devices, laboratory supplies, and other accessories used in research and clinical applications. The journal *Science* annually publishes a supplement, *Science Guide to Scientific Instruments*, that lists instruments and manufacturers. Finally, the *Encyclopedia of Instrumentation and Control* (Considine, 1971) also provides listings of instruments and equipment available. Information on available instrumentation can be obtained from texts such as *Biomedical Instrumentation and Measurements (2nd ed)* (Cromwell, Weibell, et al 1980), and Dewhurst's (1976) *An Introduction to Biomedical Instrumentation*.

Once an investigator has decided on the type of instrumentation to employ, there are issues that must be considered in the final decision as to a particular instrument. These issues include: (1) accuracy, (2) linearity, (3) hysteresis, (4) range, (5) sensitivity, and (6) reliability.

There are many potential sources of instrument inaccuracy. Cromwell and associates (1980) list operational deficiencies in design or construction, mechanical errors of meters, component drift, and temperature variations. All of these can result in measures that are invalid as data. Other sources of inaccuracy may include improper maintenance of equipment or lack of instrument calibration.

Linearity and hysteresis both involve idiosyncratic mechanical effects on measurements. Linearity involves the "amount a measurement deviates from the calibration curve" (Currier, 1984, p 186). This is a classic example of the potential for an instrumentation threat to internal validity discussed in Chapter 3. The linear instrument follows the calibration curve for the entire measurement range. The inaccurate instrument deviates from the curve for some portion of the curve. The readings for a part of the range are accurate, whereas those for another portion are not. Hysteresis refers to the difference in instrument readings that occurs when instrument readings are influenced by the direction on the scale in which the readings are taken. When a problem of hysteresis exists, for example, readings taken in ascending order on the scale will differ from readings for the same phenomenon taken in descending order.

The range and sensitivity that are necessary in equipment will, of course, depend on the type and necessary accuracy of the measures to be taken. The *combination* of range and sensitivity is also an important consideration, since differential sensitivity across the range will result in invalid data.

The reliability of instrumentation should be considered from two vantage points. The first involves the amount of time that the equipment will be functional. Clearly, the researcher cannot collect any sort of data if the equipment is broken. The second type of reliability has to do with issues discussed in Chapter 3 in terms of the stability and trustworthiness of the instrument's measurements.

The physical measures employed in a study clearly depend on the procedures of data collection. Investigators employing physical measures as dependent variables have the advantages of a plethora of available equipment and instrumentation. Because of the instrumentation available, researchers do not often find themselves in the position of being forced to develop their own instruments. On the other hand, researchers who would measure subjects' level of information, attitudes, or capabilities often find that no appropriate instrumentation is available, which brings us to the issues concerning the development and use of written instruments for data collection.

□ WRITTEN INSTRUMENTS □

As discussed in Chapter 6, data for descriptive research are often collected through the use of written surveys, questionnaires, and tests. Many such instruments have been developed and standardized. These standardized instruments are useful in that there are fewer questions about their validity and reliability and they are accompanied by norms that allow the investigator to evaluate her or his results. Because of the breadth of topics that may be covered by written instruments, however, many researchers discover that no such standardized instrument is available for their specific purposes. In this chapter we will focus on how to locate and develop written instruments, discussing such issues as test validity and the criteria to be employed in evaluating written instruments.

□ TEST VALIDITY □

In Chapter 3 we discussed the concept of validity in terms of research design in general. Test validity is a special case that applies specifically to written tests and more generally to other written data collection instruments. Like the more general case, test validity concerns the accuracy of the measures employed. We will consider three categories of test validity: (1) content validity, (2) construct validity, and (3) criterion-related validity.

Content validity concerns the representativeness or sampling adequacy of the items in the instrument. A valid test must contain measures that tap all facets of the phenomenon of interest. For example, if your instructor told you to prepare for a comprehensive final examination based on this entire text, but the actual examination consisted of questions based on only one chapter, the test would lack content validity.

In most cases the universe or population of material to be sampled is not as clearly defined as in the example above. In such cases, the researcher should attempt to first define the content as exhaustively as possible, identifying any subsets of material. Then (in either developing or evaluating an instrument) the researcher should ascertain that the subsets have been represented in the instrument.

A final concern of content validity is that the test should actually measure what it purports to measure and not something else. A questionnaire on attitudes toward health care facilities distributed to individuals with low educational levels may become in fact merely a measure of reading ability. Thus, content-valid tests measure the intended subject, and only the intended subject.

Construct validity, as used in relation to test validity, has much the same meaning as that given in our previous definition (Chapter 3). Construct validity in testing can almost be thought of as analogous to content validity, with theoretical concepts representing one universe of content. A construct-valid test exhaustively measures the various theoretical facets of a construct. The important distinction with construct validity "is its preoccupation with theory, theoretical constructs, and scientific empirical inquiry involving the testing of hypothesized relations" (Kerlinger, 1965, pp 461-462). Thus, content and construct validity in testing represent the polar extremes of a continuum ranging from the concrete to the theoretically amorphous.

There are two types of criterion-related validity: predictive and concurrent. In both cases an outside criterion is compared to the test to determine its accuracy in measuring a phenomenon. Predictive validity involves the ability of an instrument to forecast future behavior or measures. A researcher might develop a scale measuring the attitudes of patients with spinal cord injury as a predictor of eventual extent of recovery. Insofar as scores on the scale are related to level of eventual recovery, the scale would be considered valid.

Concurrent validity refers to the relationship between the instrument in question and other (validated) instruments that measure the same phenomenon. For example, a researcher who developed a new instrument to evaluate sensory processing might want to compare scores on the new instrument to scores on the Southern California Integration Tests.

Perhaps the issue of concurrent validity seems a bit puzzling. Why create redundant measures? If adequate measures of a phenomenon already exist, why bother with a new measure? Good question. New measures should represent an improvement of some sort over existing measures. In other words, the new measure should be easier for subjects to understand, or less time-consuming, or in some other way better than other instruments.

The methods of establishing test validity of an instrument depend on the type of validity that is in question. For criterion-related validity, scores are compared directly and a measure known as the correlation coefficient is calculated (see Chapter 13). The researcher can thus quantify the relationship as an aid in establishing validity.

Content and construct validity cannot be so precisely determined. There is no quantification or statistical technique to be performed. In both cases the determination of validity is essentially a judgment call. In such cases it is probably wise to seek the opinion of colleagues because the designer of an instrument is often so highly involved and so steeped in the subject as to cloud objectivity.

□ LOCATING WRITTEN INSTRUMENTS □

Before the researcher invests the time and effort needed to design a written instrument, he or she should take the time to determine whether there is an existing instrument that may be employed or modified for use. Researchers tend to be too quick to develop their own instruments, perhaps because of the apparent ease with which this task may be accomplished. Considerations of validity, reliability, and scaling aside, it is actually quite a task to develop a good questionnaire or assessment device. Therefore it is wise, when possible, to draw on the results of methodological research for proven instruments.

The search for a standardized instrument may begin in any of several places. If in the literature researchers encounter a study that employs an instrument that appears to meet the needs of their research, they may establish contact with the study's author. In such situations researchers may find themselves contributing to the standardization of an instrument by sharing their data with the form's author.

Two resources are available in the library that may aid in the process of locating appropriate measures. *Tests in Print* (Buros, 1974), and *Mental Measurements Yearbook* (Buros, ed., 1978) contain listings of tests of intelligence, development, aptitudes, and vocational interests. The yearbook contains reviews of the tests and references regarding their use. These listings also indicate the publisher of the instrument. Table 8-1 contains some of the more frequently employed standardized tests.

The various disciplines in the health sciences have differed in the extent to which specific standardized instruments have been developed. Nursing and occupational therapy research, because of their subject matter, have often employed tests that were originally developed by psychologists. In addition, occupational therapy has begun to develop unique instruments such as the Prevocational Motor Skills Inventory (Brown & Van der Bogert), Evaluation of Work Behavior (Ayres), Physical Capacities Evaluation (Smith), and the Workshop Trainee Evaluation (Trombly & Scott). Texts such as Reed's (1984) *Models of Practice in Occupational Therapy* provide sources for such tests.

TABLE 8-1 STANDARDIZED TESTS

Intelligence Tests and Developmental Scales
    Bayley Infant Scales of Development
    Vineland Social Maturity Scale
    Wechsler Adult Intelligence Scale (R)
    Stanford-Binet Intelligence Scale
Sensory Motor Tests
    Pennsylvania Bimanual Work Sample
    Minnesota Spatial Relations Test
Vocational Inventories
    Strong Vocational Interest Blank
    Kuder Preference Record
Work Samples
    Singer Vocational Evaluation System
    Talent Assessment Program

Often, however, particularly when the phenomenon of interest involves a specific situation, such as the attitudes of students toward a proposed curriculum change at a particular institution, no standardized instrument is available, and researchers must develop their own instruments. It is to this situation that we now turn.

□ DEVELOPING WRITTEN INSTRUMENTS □

Many of the issues involved in developing a good written assessment instrument are the same as for the development of interviews (see Chapter 7). Because there is no interaction between people involved in the use of written instruments, there are a number of special concerns to be addressed.

The instructions to the respondent must be stated in an extremely clear and straightforward manner. If respondents do not understand how to complete the form they may not attempt it. Worse yet, from the point of view of valid data, they might. Responses might be random and function only as noise in the data.

Directions should be given in short, clear sentences. The level of the language should be carefully selected so that respondents will be familiar with the terminology employed. The researcher should be careful not to talk down to subjects, however, since this might create resentment. Instructions should be respectful and polite. In this same vein, the instructions should close with a statement of thanks for the cooperation of the subjects. (A pleasant side effect of this practice is that it tends to increase the return rate of forms.)

Directions for each type of item should be specific. How many alternatives should be chosen? If asking subjects to rank items, should #1 be the best or the worst? Whenever possible, provide an example of each type of item with the response indicated and explained. Often, a short demonstration is clearer than a long explanation.

The entire instrument should be short. Written instruments should only be used to obtain information not obtainable through other sources. Subjects become bored with longer forms or may simply not complete the form at all. Longer forms may be acceptable if the issue is extremely interesting and salient to subjects.

The form should be laid out in such a way as to facilitate understanding and completion of items. Conservation of paper is unwise; crowding items may confuse respondents. Generally, a list of alternatives such as that shown in Table 8-2a is clearer than the form shown in 8-2b.

The ordering of questions should follow the same principles as the ordering of interview questions. The first questions should be general and interesting to subjects. Items should be organized into logical groups on

TABLE 8-2 FORMATTING QUESTIONNAIRE ITEMS

a. Please indicate the number of times in the past year a family member has required medical treatment:
   (a) treatment not required _____
   (b) 1 – 5 times _____
   (c) 6 – 10 times _____
   (d) 11 or more times _____
b. Please indicate the number of times in the past year a family member has required medical treatment: (a) treatment not required _____; (b) 1 – 5 times _____; (c) 6 – 10 times _____; (d) 11 or more times _____

related topics. Questions on sensitive or threatening material should appear toward the end of the form. This will help reduce the amount of data that will be lost if a respondent refuses to complete the form. It also allows the respondent more time to become comfortable with the process, which ideally will reduce the possibility of respondent refusals.

It should be clear to respondents what they are to do with the completed forms. If they are to be mailed to the researcher, an addressed, stamped envelope should be included. It is often wise to provide the respondents with a time frame for return (e.g., within a week or by a specific date) to prevent respondents from forgetting to complete the form. If the respondent is to complete the form in the presence of the researcher, it is a considerate gesture to provide an envelope or folder into which the respondent may place the completed forms. This formality appears to emphasize the importance of the data collection process to respondents who in turn feel more valued (and often become more cooperative).

The process of eliciting initial cooperation and ensuring return of the research instrument is usually accomplished through the use of separate cover and follow-up letters. As mentioned in Chapter 6, the cover letter often represents the first contact between researcher and subject and creates an impression in the mind of the subject that may well influence subsequent cooperation. The cover letter should be formal and polite. It should outline the project, establish the professional affiliation of the researcher, and request participation in the study. It should also explain how the completed form is to be returned to the investigator, often indicating a time frame during which response is desired. Finally, the letter should express gratitude to subjects for their time and cooperation.

Return rates for completed questionnaires are frequently quite low. In order to increase returns, the investigator should employ a follow-up contact—often a letter. After the lapse of an interval of time from the initial mailing, a follow-up letter to nonrespondents reminding them of the project may well stimulate some subjects to respond. More than three follow-up contacts to the initial group of subjects is generally considered to be wasteful of the researcher's time. If the response continues to be extremely low, the investigator should examine the instrument or cover letter for explanations of the poor showing and consider choosing an additional sample for the study.

Question Format

Ideally, questionnaires should contain a combination of open-ended and closed questions. Open-ended questions were discussed in Chapter 7. We turn now to a discussion of closed questions.

In closed questions, respondents are faced with a set of fixed alternatives from which to choose. Subjects are thus limited as to their potential responses. There are both advantages and disadvantages to such a format.

The advantages of closed questions primarily involve ease of administration and tabulation. As subjects merely mark responses and need not take the time to write out a long response, more items of information may be collected. This very ease, however, creates some problems and may mask the existence of others.

The temptation to increase the number of items may be irresistible to the researcher, resulting in an over-long form. More seriously, the semi-mechanical nature of the responses to closed ended questions may mask the fact that there is a lack of communication between researcher and respondent. The researcher may not have communicated clearly in the item or the respondent may not understand either the question or the format. But, as long as answers are indicated, there is no way of knowing if this problem exists. This is one reason it is wise to include a few open-ended questions to check for clarity.

Another advantage of the closed question is that in written questionnaires (as opposed to interviews) this format facilitates response to threatening material. Whereas a subject may not respond to a threatening open-ended question, the inclusion of response categories appears to reassure respondents not only that the behavior or attitude in question is acceptable, but also that there is an acceptable range of responses.

The disadvantages of the closed question format are that it limits the range of potential response, creates an attitude or opinion with the question, and limits the researcher's ability to judge the importance or salience of the question to the respondent. The response categories must be exhaustive of the possible responses to the question. If they are not, the researcher loses information, since respondents may indicate the closest response to their actual opinion or behavior. Subjects may also resent being forced to choose categories rather than respond freely.

The ability to simply mark a response category may also result in the artificial creation of an opinion or attitude. When faced with an issue never before considered, the subject can choose from a ready-made set of possible responses without having to consider the issue. This property of the closed question format also obscures the relevance or salience of the question to subjects. Subjects' opinions on zebra hunting in Manhattan would weigh equally with their responses on such potentially emotional issues as disposal of nuclear waste, euthanasia, or abortion. It cannot be determined from the closed question whether the respondent even possessed an opinion or attitude on the subject before being asked about it. The disadvantages of closed questions can be minimized through the addition of open-ended questions to the form and through careful attention to the construction of items.

Item Wording

The single most important issue in item wording is clarity. All other concerns revolve around whether the subject correctly understands the question. Clarity involves both structure and content of items. The items (both question—also referred to as the *stem*—and responses) should consist of short, simple sentences. The language should employ the vernacular and be within the reading ability of respondents. Statements should avoid the use of double-negative constructions.

Content issues revolve around interpretation. Items should tap a single issue. Nonspecific or overly complex statements leave respondents at a loss as to the meaning of the response alternatives. Researchers should be careful to define terms and not use ambiguous generic terms. Differential definition of terms may well influence respondent response. For example, Labaw (1980), found the term "family planning" variously interpreted as meaning birth control, financial planning, and planning for family outings. This misunderstanding resulted in systematic bias, because women were more likely to understand the term as applying to birth control and men to financial planning.

Response Formats

The clearly stated stem in a closed question should be followed by equally clearly stated alternatives. Various types of formats and scales may be employed to collect responses. The general rule that applies to all formats is that response choices should exhaust the range of possible responses and should be mutually exclusive so that a respondent is clear as to the one appropriate category for his or her response.

Probably the most commonly employed response format is some variation of multiple choice. The simplest form is the dichotomous yes/no format. Not everyone will be able to respond to this forced choice, however, so often a third category of "don't know" or "no opinion" is included. When subjects are being presented with several alternatives, the number of categories should be kept limited. Subjects may have trouble with more than five alternatives—especially on attitude or opinion rather than behavioral topics. The question of including the "no opinion" option is the subject of some controversy and is discussed later in the chapter.

Checklists provide subjects with a list of behaviors or attitudes, asking them to indicate the ones that they do or do not perform or approve of. In such simple form, a checklist actually represents a different format of the forced-choice dichotomous multiple-choice question. Checklists can be expanded into matrix form if the number of alternative columns to be selected is expanded as illustrated in Table 8-3.

In some cases subjects may be asked to rank items along some criterion such as importance or approval. In such cases it is extremely important to hold the number of alternatives to be ranked below ten. Any more items tend to confuse subjects. If possible, the ideal maximum number of items to rank should be held at five or six (Orlich, 1978).

Agree _____   _____   _____   _____   _____ Disagree

A number of scales have been developed for the collection of data. The simplest form of scale is the bipolar scale as seen above. Subjects indicate their position on a continuum between bipolar opposites such as agree/disagree. The bipolar scale represents an expansion of the dichotomous multiple choice response as now subjects indicate the extent of agreement/disagreement through the placement of their response.

The number of alternative spaces between the poles has been the subject of much discussion with the controversy centering around whether to use an odd or an even number of spaces. The use of an odd number creates a "no opinion" midline possible response whereas the use of an even

---

TABLE 8-3 EXAMPLES OF CHECKLIST AND MATRIX FORMATS

Checklist
Indicate any of the following you have experienced in the last year:
Fatigue _____
Headaches _____
Nosebleeds _____
Blurred vision _____
Insomnia _____

Matrix
Indicate the number of times within the last year you have experienced each of the following symptoms:

	Never	1–5 times	6–10 times	11+ times
Fatigue	_____	_____	_____	_____
Headaches	_____	_____	_____	_____
Nosebleeds	_____	_____	_____	_____
Blurred vision	_____	_____	_____	_____
Insomnia	_____	_____	_____	_____

number of response spaces forces the subject to take a position. This discussion is analogous to that centering on whether to include a "no opinion" option in a multiple-choice format. The concern is that some subjects will choose only this option—which basically represents a non-response. Advocates of the even number of spaces prefer to force an opinion and thus ensure data. Proponents of the odd number of spaces ("no opinion") argue that it is poor research practice to create data. If subjects wish not to respond for whatever reason, that should be accepted, they argue. There is no clear, compelling argument to settle the dispute. The decision as to the number of scale positions is left to the instrument author.

The Semantic Differential Scale (Osgood, Suci, Tannenbaum, 1957) employs the bipolar scale format using pairs of adjectives as the end points—for example, acceptable/not acceptable, passive/active. Generally there are three dimensions into which these adjective pairs can be categorized—the evaluative dimension (good/bad), the potency dimension (strong/weak), and the activity dimension (fast/slow). The authors suggest the use of adjective pair items that tap all three dimensions.

In each pair of adjectives, one word will represent a more socially desirable option. When constructing a semantic differential scale, it is wise to alternate the side of the form of the "better" response. This strategy prevents subjects from simply marking down one side of the scale—or if they do, it makes it clear that responses were not carefully thought through.

The Likert scale (developed by psychologist Rensis Likert) provides a scale of agreement/disagreement in a matrix-style format. Again the number of positions between the endpoints enables or disallows the "no opinion" option. In creating a Likert-scaled form it is wise to randomly alternate positive and negative wording of the items. This again forces the subject to read each item more carefully and reduces the probability of a response bias.

The Guttman or cumulative scale is the most difficult to construct. Alternatives are constructed so that agreement with a third alternative also indicates agreement with the first two alternatives. Because many issues make construction of such alternatives quite difficult, Guttman scales are not often used.

□ EVALUATING INSTRUMENTS □

Having either found a ready-made instrument or having constructed an original, the researcher needs a set of criteria for use in evaluating the instrument. The ideal instrument can be proved valid and reliable. In the absence of such proof, Orlich (1978) suggests the following criteria: (1) parsimony, (2) specificity, (3) simplicity, (4) lack of bias, and (5) manageability. The form should be as short as possible to be consistent with collecting the necessary data and should be clear and understandable to subjects.

Belson (1981) suggests that a good instrument will:

Avoid:
    Loading up the question with a lot of different or defining terms
    Offering long alternatives (as possible answers to a question)
    Using words that are not the usual working tools of the respondent
    Using words that mean something different if partly misheard
    Giving the respondent a difficult task to perform
    Giving the respondent a task that calls for a major memory effort
    Offering alternatives that could both be true
Beware:
    The strong tendency of respondents to answer questions about their behavior in terms of what they usually do, as distinct from what they did in fact do
    The use of the qualifying clause, especially at the end of a question
    The tendency of respondents to start answering a question as soon as they have heard enough to start formulating a reply

The data obtained through the use of a written instrument is only as good as the instrument itself. Pretesting of constructed instruments will help ensure their validity. Careful researchers devote a great deal of time and attention to the development of written data collection instruments.

□ RESPONSE BIAS □

Some subjects show tendencies to respond to written questionnaires in set patterns that may have little to do with either the reality of attitudes or behaviors or even the content of the instrument. These patterned behaviors are known as response sets or response biases. Knowledge of the more common sets may allow the researcher, through construction of the instrument, to minimize the effect of such biases or to at least recognize the presence of such biased data. The most commonly encountered sets include: (1) acquiescence or negativity, (2) social desirability, (3) extreme responses, (4) halo effects, and (5) systematic severity or leniency of ratings.

In the case of the acquiescence or negativity biases we see the Yea-sayers and the Nay-sayers. Some people will agree with every statement, regardless of content. The negativity bias involves the person who will disagree with every statement.

The social desirability bias involves the subjects' natural desire to be respectable. Society differentially approves or disapproves behaviors. Those who show the social desirability bias answer in the socially approved direction. A scale was developed by Crowne and Marlowe (1964) that measures the tendency to this bias. In the case of a topic that might be heavily influenced by social desirability, the investigator might consider administering the Crown-Marlowe scale and using the score as a covariate in an analysis of covariance (see Chapter 12).

Some standardized tests have built-in subscales that measure for social desirability. The Minnesota Multiphasic Personality Inventory (MMPI) contains a scale (called the *L* scale) based on a group of items that make the examinee appear in a favorable light, but are unlikely to be truthfully answered in the favorable direction (Anastasi, 1968). Such subscales allow the investigator to recognize the potential for bias in the data.

Berg (1955, 1957, 1959, 1961) identified a responses bias referred to as "deviation." This is the tendency of the respondent to choose the most extreme available option, regardless of the direction of the deviation, or the content of the measure. Such data are clearly invalid.

Halo effects are seen when ratings are requested of various aspects of an object and one characteristic affects the ratings of other (supposedly independent) characteristics. For example, ratings of intelligence and competence will be higher for those who are physically attractive. The reverse effect may also be seen, where one negative factor or characteristic tends to drag other ratings down.

The final biases may represent subjects' personality characteristics. Some people rate everything severely, almost never employing the more positive ratings. Others reverse the bias, and all their ratings of anything exhibit extreme leniency.

What can the researcher do about response bias? Not a lot. Fortunately the phenomenon is not particularly common. Forms may be constructed that upset the patterns and render such sets difficult. Or subscales may be constructed and criteria preset for deletion of responses from the data set. Eliminating forms that "appear to show bias" *after* data have been collected is not acceptable. Such a practice smacks of eliminating data that are unfavorable to the hypothesis (that is, cheating). The best the investigator can do after the fact is to write such bias off to noise and hope that the effect under consideration is strong enough to appear through the static provided by the biased responses.

□ SUMMARY □

Data for health-science research can be collected through the use of physical instrumentation known as hardware and through written instruments such as surveys and questionnaires. Physical hardware allows for phenomena such as joint motion or lung capacity to be measured and is usually commercially designed and constructed. Several publications serve to keep researchers informed of the varieties of hardware available for research. In employing and selecting physical instrumentation, the investigator must be conscious of such issues as accuracy, linearity, hysteresis, range, sensitivity, and reliability of the equipment.

Numerous standardized written data collection surveys and questionnaires are also available to the researcher. Because of the specificity of research on such issues as attitudes and opinions, however, many researchers choose to develop their own data collection forms. Although seemingly a simple task, the careful development of an appropriate questionnaire involves questions of test validity, attention to question format and wording, and the selection of the most appropriate form of response format. All of these issues affect such crucial research concerns as subjects' comprehension of the task and willingness to complete the form. Proper design of written instruments can also aid in disrupting the tendency of subjects to demonstrate various response biases or tendencies to respond in patterned, unthinking ways.

□ KEY TERMS □

hardware	checklists
linearity	matrix
hysteresis	semantic differential
range	Likert scale
test validity	Guttman scale (cumulative scale)
content validity	response bias
construct validity	social desirability bias
criterion-related validity	acquiescence bias
concurrent validity	negativity bias
predictive validity	halo effect
closed questions	deviation bias
multiple choice	

9

Design Pitfalls

- □ *Experimental Bias*
  - □ *Experimenter Bias*
  - □ *Instrument Bias*
  - □ *Subject Effects*
- □ *Demand Characteristics*
- □ *Research Ethics*

Before we begin to discuss methods of analyzing research data, it is essential that we pause and consider some very important issues. Research results are only useful in terms of generalizability and advancement of a discipline to the extent that they present a distortion-free, unbiased picture of the phenomenon under examination. Although the use of good research design will help minimize distortion, there are several types of bias that may still affect the data. In this chapter we will discuss biases introduced by experimenters, by research instruments, and by subjects themselves.

An extremely important concern in the research process is the protection of the rights and welfare of subjects. We will examine the various ethical dilemmas inherent in the research process and discuss solutions that the various disciplines have adopted.

□ EXPERIMENTAL BIAS □

Each one of the component parts of the research process has the potential to introduce bias into the research data. Experimenters who painstakingly control the design of their studies may inadvertently either elicit specific

responses from subjects or selectively perceive the desired effects in subjects' behavior. The data collection instrument may elicit biased responses
through either content or format. Finally, subjects themselves, through
their responses, may introduce systematic bias into data even above and
beyond the response sets discussed in Chapter 8.

Experimenter Bias

Although there have been unfortunate cases where investigators have deliberately falsified or influenced research results, the great majority of scientists are honest and ethical in their conduct of research. We shall
consider, then, only those sources of influence that the experimenter may
introduce unintentionally into subjects' behaviors and responses. Deliberate attempts to control research outcomes, needless to say, are morally
reprehensible and scientifically inexcusable.

The experimenter may introduce unintentional bias through interactions with either the data or the subjects themselves. Whenever the experimenter is responsible for data collection through such means as
interviews or observations, the process of selective perception may bias
results.

Most people believe that what they observe of the world around them
accurately reflects the contents of the world. There is ample evidence to
show that this may simply not be so. Social psychologist Donald Campbell
(1967) has advanced a theory to explain perceptive distortion which he
refers to as the "downstream periscope" model of perception.

When we visually perceive the world, the information on our perceptions is passed through the brain and processed in the occipital lobe.
Campbell argues that because the information passes through the "asso-
ciative tracts" of the brain before we ever become aware of the stimulus,
unconscious alteration of the information has already taken place by the
time the stimulus becomes conscious. This alteration serves to tailor the
input to fit our preconceived notions and stereotypes. Thus biasing occurs
at a preconscious, unintentional level. Research has shown that perceptions of such basic characteristics as competence and even physical attrac-
tiveness may be biased by stereotypes and prejudices. Thus an observer/
experimenter who firmly believes in his or her research hypothesis may
prove to be an unreliable observer of behaviors.

Another psychologist (Weick, 1968) categorized types of observer bias.
One such effect is the tendency of observers to create clear-cut categories
of observations. Similarities between categories are underestimated and
differences are exaggerated. Observers also tend to assimilate observations
into categories with which they are familiar, thus perhaps artificially reducing the variability in the data.

These same cognitive biasing factors may play a role in the scoring of
written data when the scorer is aware of the research hypothesis, espe-

cially if the treatment status of the subject is known. Knowledge of the subject's category membership may invoke any expectations or hopes that the scorer may have about the responses the subject "should" be making.

The potential for experimenter bias is illuminated by the results of research conducted by Rosenthal (1966). Rosenthal's investigations have uncovered a number of ways in which experimenters' behaviors may influence subject responses. In order for all subjects to be exposed to standardized stimuli, experimenters should treat all subjects identically. Rosenthal found that male experimenters behave toward subjects in a friendlier manner than do female experimenters and that all experimenters are more likely to smile at female subjects.

In and of themselves these behavioral differences might not seem very alarming, since there are many dependent variables that might not be affected by subjects' mood or rapport with the experimenter. Unfortunately, Rosenthal has demonstrated that experimenters tend to provide cues to subjects about expected behaviors. These cues are quite subtle, but most effective in influencing not only the behavior of human subjects, who might be expected to be sensitive to experimenters' behaviors, but also the behavior of animal subjects.

In a study on learning in rats, experimenters were told by Rosenthal and Lanson (1964) that their rats represented strains that had been especially bred to be either "bright" or "dull." Actually the rats had been randomly assigned to the two groups. As predicted, "bright" rats acquired new behaviors faster than the "dull" rats. Similar effects have been found in learning studies with other animals, including planaria! In addition, the phenomenon of expectancy effects has been demonstrated in studies involving "human learning, psychophysical judgment, reaction time, inkblot tests, structured laboratory interviews and person perception" (Carlsmith, Ellsworth, and Aronson, 1976, p 293).

If expectancy effects are so pervasive and so potentially distorting of experimental results, what steps can be taken to reduce the problem? A series of techniques have been developed that involve keeping the person who might provide the expectancy cues ignorant of the cues that would support the research hypothesis. These are known as "blind" techniques.

When the research involves observation of behaviors, two techniques may be employed. The observers may be kept blind to the hypotheses of the study altogether: Observers cannot communicate what they themselves do not know. An alternative technique allows the observers to learn the experimental hypotheses but keeps them blind to the treatment status of subjects during the observations: An observer who does not know whether a subject represents the treatment or the control condition will not know which set of cues to give. This same technique of keeping the experimenter blind to the subjects' status is also effective in reducing bias in scoring written protocols or ratings.

The most elaborate blind technique is known as the double blind and involves several layers of research personnel. As it is somewhat esoteric, perhaps it is best explained through the use of an example.

Dr. X has just perfected (he hopes) a drug that will eliminate pain. Because he is aware of the potential strength of expectancy effects, he decides to test the drug's effectiveness employing the double blind technique. First he manufactures a tablet that looks identical to the experimental drug. This tablet may consist of either an inert substance (a placebo—to be discussed later in this chapter) or an analgesic such as aspirin to serve as a baseline. He labels bottles of his experimental drug as "A" and the non-treatment containers are labeled "B". He chooses samples of subjects (of course using appropriate techniques) then hires his research staff.

He tells his research staff he is performing comparative tests of drugs A and B. At this point he makes no further disclosures. His research staff assigns subjects to either condition A or condition B then prepares the medication for subjects (identical doses of identical tablets). The tablets are administered to patients by nurses who are not given any information about the study.

Thus, the researcher is insulated from subjects by two layers of staff. The first layer does not know which drug is which or what the difference between the drugs might be. Therefore they cannot in any way communicate expectations to the nurses, who have no expectations to communicate to their patients. When such a technique is used, it is virtually impossible to cite expectancy effects as the source for any observed differences in pain reduction.

Such elaborate techniques may not be necessary, of course. But whenever expectancy cues from experimenters may influence outcome measures it is best to provide as little basis for cues as possible.

Instrument Effects

The actual instruments used to collect dependent measures may serve as a source of bias. As discussed in Chapters 3 and 8, acceptable data can only be collected with reliable instruments that have been proven valid. The instrument must measure what it purports to measure, and the scaling of the measure must be standardized across the range of measurement. If the instrumentation does not fulfil these requirements, it poses a threat to internal validity and may seriously hamper the interpretation of experimental results.

In addition to these basic concerns, various types of research have inherent sources of potential bias. In historical research the data consist of historical documents, relics, and testimony of witnesses. A primary source of bias in this type of research involves the availability of these data. If all possible sources of data were available to the investigator, bias would be less of a concern. This is seldom the case, however. When only partial records are available, the researcher must seriously consider the question of why this particular set of data has survived. The records may be incomplete simply because of limitations on space or funds or, a more sinister case, because of deliberate bias in favor (or against) a particular source or type of data. Imagine, for example, a future historical researcher considering attitudes toward abortion in the 1980s who could uncover only documents from the "right-to-life" movement rather than having access to documents from all the various points of view.

In interviews or written questionnaires the format and the content may introduce bias. Questions or items that "lead" the subject make very clear the desired responses. However, such obvious (and ethically objectionable) practices may not be the only way in which subjects gain cues. Knowledge of the institutional affiliation of the experimenter gained from the letterhead or return address may provide sufficient cues to the subjects. A questionnaire on attitudes toward socialized medicine would probably yield different subject responses if the responsible agency was identified as the American Socialist Party as opposed to the American Medical Association.

Subject Effects

Subjects themselves may introduce bias both through who they are and how they behave. The problem of selection bias is discussed in Chapters 3 through 6 as a serious potential threat to internal validity. This problem is particularly severe when subjects are volunteers. Such self-selection may bias the results of a study toward characteristics shared by subjects that are irrelevant to (or distracting from) the variables of interest. Researchers should be alert to the problems presented by self-selection both in volunteerism and in subjects who actually complete a research study (independent of initial method of selection). If there are different rates of attrition from the study based on subject characteristics, results may be biased. Methods for assessing the extent of nonequivalence in final samples are discussed in Chapter 13.

Subject responses and behaviors may represent sources of bias in certain methods of data collection. As has been mentioned, self-report measures are more susceptible to bias than are behavioral measures (when the subject and not the observer is being considered as the source of potential bias). If the topic involves reporting self-incriminating behaviors (such as illegal drug usage) subjects may lie to protect themselves. Subjects may also lie about demographic characteristics to protect their self-image— e.g., falsifying age or income. Also, subjects may exhibit any of the response biases discussed in Chapter 8 (acquiescence bias, the tendency to provide extreme responses, to provide socially desirable responses, to provide lenient or severe judgments, and halo effects).

□ DEMAND CHARACTERISTICS □

As discussed above, subjects tend to be very sensitive to experimenters in reading behavioral cues. The term "demand characteristics" was coined by Martin Orne (1962) to describe the phenomenon in which subjects are so anxious to oblige the researcher that they behave so appropriately as subjects that they exhibit atypical behaviors. As the term *expectancy* deals with the experimenter's side of the phenomenon, the term *demand characteristics* focuses attention on the response of subjects.

Orne's (1962) classic study involved having subjects add columns of numbers on sheets of paper then tear the paper into 32 pieces. Orne wanted to see how long subjects would continue with this obviously pointless behavior. Subjects continued for up to several hours before stopping!

Orne has argued that entire lines of research may be contaminated with demand characteristics. In particular he has pointed a finger at the sensory deprivation research conducted in the early 1960s and dropped because of alleged serious effects on subjects.

Typical sensory deprivation research involved floating subjects in body-temperature salt water in a tank that was sound- and light-proof. Such studies were conducted in hospitals and medical schools, subjects were given pre-experimental physical examinations, and asked to sign releases absolving the experimenter of any liability for harm the subject might receive. Trays of emergency medical equipment were in full sight outside the tank and subjects were shown the "panic button" which would summon the immediate attention of the experimenter. Subjects were warned of possible symptoms that might result from sensory deprivation. Not surprisingly, a large number used the panic button and reported symptoms from the experimenters' lists.

Orne pointed out that the entire situation had been presented as potentially dangerous and that subjects had even been provided scripts for their responses. To make his point he set up a sensory deprivation experiment in which subjects spent time in a room equipped with a table and chair, food, water, and an arithmetic task. For half the subjects the procedures for the standard sensory deprivation experiments were duplicated, down to the releases and the panic button. For the other half, such threatening cues were removed. A significant proportion of the treatment group reported the same symptoms as the real sensory deprivation subjects—including hallucinations. So a very real question remains about the original research. It is quite possible that all effects had to do with instructional sets provided to subjects. It is interesting to note that a recent fad industry capitalized on the concept of the sensory deprivation chamber to develop small-scale sensory deprivation units billed as relaxation chambers for which individuals were willing to pay for the alleged effects in order to "unwind."

Researchers must be extremely sensitive to the possibility that they may be providing subjects with cues to desired responses. There are several steps investigators can take to counteract the potential effects of demand characteristics. Behavioral measures may be employed. Because these are more difficult for the subject to control, they may be less easily affected. The subject may also deliberately be given a false hypothesis by the experimenter. If behaviors conform to this fictional hypothesis, demand characteristics must be considered a problem. As this solution involves deceiving subjects, there are ethical issues to be considered.

Probably the most commonly employed technique to counter demand characteristics is the use of the placebo. Essentially a placebo is a nontreatment disguised so the subject believes he or she has received some treatment. In drug effectiveness studies, if subjects know they are testing a new pain reliever, a certain percentage will report pain relief even if given an inert substance instead of the drug.

In a placebo study several groups receive identical treatment, but only one receives the actual drug. If the drug is administered by capsule, control subjects receive identical capsules. If the drug is administered through injection, controls receive injections of saline solution. If subjects report effectiveness for the inert substance, demand characteristics may provide the explanation. The use of double blind procedures combined with the use of a placebo (as described earlier in the chapter) effectively counter expectancy effects and demand characteristics.

□ RESEARCH ETHICS □

A primary concern of the ethical researcher is the protection of subjects—both animal and human—from harm. Harm has been defined to include physical or mental stress and danger.

Unfortunately, the line between appropriate research and unethical treatment of subjects is not always clear. How much danger to subjects is too much? What if the potential benefits to mankind are overwhelmingly large, but testing involves what some would label cruelty to animal subjects? Because zealous researchers may lack objectivity and because disciplines and institutions are responsible for the behaviors of their constituents, both disciplines and institutions have established guidelines for ethical behavior. Institutions have committees that review research proposals by employees and must approve the proposal before the research may be undertaken or extra-mural sources of funds contacted. Funding agencies demand such institutional ethics approval as a part of the grant proposal.

Various disciplines have established formal codes for ethical behavior for both research and clinical practice and have developed systems of sanctions against individuals who do not adhere to the guidelines.

The American Psychological Association and the American Medical Association publish detailed monographs on ethical standards. Other disciplines, such as physical therapy and occupational therapy, publish articles in their major journals (Michels, 1976). Many of these guidelines are based on the World Medical Association's Declaration of Helsinki (Table 9.1).

There are basically three important areas in which the rights of subjects must be protected. These pertain to (1) their inclusion as subjects, (2) the privacy of their behavior as subjects, and (3) their general well-being. Subjects' decision to participate in research must be entirely voluntary. Subjects must feel completely free to decline to participate without fear of any reprisals. From this standpoint the use of prisoners as subjects, or even the use of classes of students in a professor's research, is questionable.

Before participation, the subject must give informed consent. This consists in signing a document that states that the subject understands the study, is participating voluntarily, and understands his or her rights as a subject. The concept of informed consent becomes somewhat murky when research is conducted on children or persons of limited mental capacity. In such cases consent is obtained from the parent or guardian. But in such cases, is the actual subject's inclusion voluntary? Or informed? Subjects must know that they may refuse to participate, refuse to provide any part of the data, and may leave the study at any point without prejudice.

A serious issue surrounding informed consent is the employment of deception on the part of the researcher. As just discussed, there are some very practical reasons why subjects should not know too much about a study in advance. Researchers want to avoid the problems of bias. This issue is often dealt with through obtaining an informed consent at the outset of the study which involves the cover story or deception employed in the research. Then after data have been collected, the subject is debriefed—that is, the real purpose and hypotheses of the study are presented. At that point subjects are offered the option of refusing to allow the researcher to use the data that have been provided. True informed consent advises the subject of the rights and risks associated with participation in the study.

The privacy of subjects must be maintained in ethical research. The identity of subjects should be kept confidential, as should the data obtained from any one individual. One way to ensure confidentiality is to remove any identifying information from the data. In cases where it might be necessary to retain identification (e.g., to match pre- and post-tests), subjects can be assigned code numbers, which are used on data forms. In any publication resulting from the research, subjects should not be identifiable as individuals. If a researcher might wish to share data such as videotapes with colleagues, a release must be obtained from the patient. In

DECLARATION OF HELSINKI

I. Basic Principles

1. Clinical research must conform to the moral and scientific principles that justify medical research and should be based on laboratory and animal experiments or other scientifically established facts.
2. Clinical research should be conducted only by scientifically qualified persons and under the supervision of a qualified medical man.
3. Clinical research cannot legitimately be carried out unless the importance of the objective is in proprotion to the inherent risk to the subject.
4. Every clinical research project should be preceded by careful assessment of inherent risk in comparison to foreseeable benefits to the subject or to others.
5. Special caution should be exercised by the doctor in performing clinical research in which the personality of the subject is liable to be altered by drugs or experimental procedure.

II. Clinical Research Combined with Professional Care

1. In the treatment of the sick person, the doctor must be free to use a new therapeutic measure, if in his judgment it offers hope of saving life, reestablishing health, or alleviating suffering.

    If at all possible, consistent with patient psychology, the doctor should obtain the patient's freely given consent after the patient has been given a full explanation. In case of legal incapacity, consent should also be procured from the legal guardian; in case of physical incapacity the permission of the legal guardian replaces that of the patient.
2. The doctor can combine clinical research with professional care, the objective being the acquisition of new medical knowledge, only to the extent that clinical research is justified by its therapeutic value for the patient.

III. Non-Therapeutic Clinical Research

1. In the purely scientific application of clinical research carried out on a human being, it is the duty of the doctor to remain the protector of the life and health of that person on whom clinical research is being carried out.
2. The nature, the purpose and the risk of clinical research must be explained to the subject by the doctor.
3a. Clinical research on a human being cannot be undertaken without his free consent after he has been informed; if he is legally incompetent, the consent of the legal guardian should be procured.
3b. The subject of clinical research should be in such a mental, physical and legal state as to be able to exercise fully his power of choice.
3c. Consent should, as a rule, be obtained in writing. However, the responsibility for clinical research always remains with the research worker, it never falls on the subject even after consent is obtained.
4a. The investigator must respect the right of each individual to safeguard his personal integrity, especially if the subject is in a dependent relationship to the investigator.
4b. At any time during the course of clinical research the subject or his guardian should be free to withdraw permission for research to be continued.

    The investigator or the investigating team should discontinue the research if in his or their judgment, it may, if continued, be harmful to the individual.

other words, through anonymity and confidentiality of response the subject's privacy is to be respected.

Protecting the well-being of subjects covers several areas. First, subjects must only be employed in legitimate scientific research conducted by competent professionals. Subjects must not be exposed to any risks without sufficient justification. The subject must be informed of and understand any risks whatever involved in the research. The researcher must terminate either the individual session or the research study in its entirety if it becomes clear that the initial assessment of risk was understated or if the risks being taken cannot be justified by the potential gains associated with the research.

Subjects have a right to information about the outcome of any research in which they have been involved. This involves both debriefing after research sessions and communication of results by the researcher at the end of the study.

Research in the behavioral and health sciences would be seriously hampered if human and animal subjects were unavailable. To preserve the right to employ human subjects, investigators have the obligation to protect the rights and dignity of their subjects. Subjects are not annoying means to the important end of the researcher's data. Subjects are essential to the research process and should be accorded the appropriate respect.

□ SUMMARY □

Bias, or distortion, may be introduced into research findings from several sources. Experimenters may selectively perceive or interpret behaviors or responses or may even inadvertently supply subjects with "correct" responses. Expectancy effects have been found even with such lower organisms as planaria. In establishing the data collection procedures the experimenter may establish "demand characteristics" that influence subjects' responses. Techniques to prevent such bias often involve so-called "blind" techniques in which the person who actually collects the data is kept ignorant of research hypotheses and subject condition and therefore cannot communicate this information to subjects. Subjects themselves may introduce bias through their expectancies. Use of such techniques as placebos and deception reduces the risk of these effects. The instruments employed for data collection may also introduce bias. Reliable, valid instruments help ensure unbiased data.

The ethical conduct of research is a serious concern for the scientific community. Subjects must be protected from physical and psychological harm. Subjects must participate only after giving informed consent; their privacy, anonymity, and confidentiality must be protected, and their general well-being assured. The various disciplines have evolved formal codes governing the ethical conduct of research and clinical practice.

□ KEY TERMS □

experimental bias
"downstream periscope"
observer bias
experimenter bias
expectancy effects
"blind" techniques
placebo

instrument effects
subject effects
demand characteristics
research ethics
deception
informed consent
debriefing

10

Descriptive Statistics

□ *Central Tendency*
  □ *The Mean*
  □ *The Median*
  □ *The Mode*
□ *Variability*
  □ *The Range*
  □ *Standard Deviation*
  □ *The Variance*

Once you have collected your data you are faced with a set of numbers out of which you must make some sense. Particularly if you have a large data set you will wish to find ways to summarize the information. Just as a summary of a novel contains enough information to allow you to follow the story but loses almost all of the detail, so it is with summarizing data. Whenever you choose to reduce your data set, you will lose some information.

As we move through the various ways to summarize your data, we will make use of a hypothetical data set to illustrate our points. This set of scores represents a set of raw, unsorted data.

9, 12, 17, 8, 10, 16, 13, 15, 17, 11, 8, 14, 15, 11, 14, 17

The most basic form of data summarizing is re-arranging the data into what is known as an array. This simply involves reordering the data from the lowest to the highest score. Such an arrangement allows you to see the distance from the top to the bottom score and the distribution of scores across the range. The above data set displayed as an array would appear as:

8, 8, 9, 10, 11, 11, 12, 13, 14, 14, 15, 15, 16, 17, 17, 17

As you can see, an array does make more intuitive sense than a raw data set. If you have many scores, however, even with an array your data will still be hard to understand. The human mind can only comfortably handle conceptually between five and nine pieces of data (± 7). So the next step is to reduce the data array into groupings, or classes. There are various ways to decide on the number of classes to use. Generally you should choose between five and ten classes of equal size (width) that cover the entire span of the range of data scores.

Or, you can decide in advance on some arbitrary number of classes. If you do, your first step is to find the range of the data. The range is calculated by subtracting the lowest score from the highest score in your data. That gives you the distance between your scores, but since we want to know the number of data points (since the data we have are nominal in form, even though they consist of numbered scores rather than category names) we take the range and add 1.

For our data set, $(17 - 8) + 1 = 10$. If we've decided on five classes, each class should contain two scores. Suppose our scores ranged from 7 to 17? Then, $(17 - 7) + 1 = 11$. If we still want five classes, our division no longer comes out. Since we can't have 2.5 scores in a class, and if we used two scores per class we would not account for all scores, we always round up (even when the decimal is less than .5). Scores are indivisible units, so anything more than one whole score is rounded up to the next value.

Rounding our result, then, we find we have three scores per class. We would then span 3 × 5 or 15 scores. But we only have 11! We divide the overlap evenly at both ends. For our data set our first class would include scores from 5 to 7, our last class scores from 17 to 19.

The number of scores in the class is referred to as the class width. The highest and lowest scores are the class limits. As you can see from Table 10.1, for our data set the class width is 2.

TABLE 10-1 FREQUENCY DISTRIBUTIONS

Class	Boundaries	Class Mark	f	Relative f	Cumulative f
8–9	7.5–9.5	8.5	3	.1875	3
10–11	9.5–11.5	10.5	3	.1875	6
12–13	11.5–13.5	12.5	2	.1250	8
14–15	13.5–15.5	14.5	4	.2500	12
16–17	15.5–17.5	16.5	4	.2500	16
			16	1.0000	

Now that we've divided the range into categories, we sort our scores. Because numbers represent continuous measures, we need to establish cut-off points or boundaries between our classes. To do this, we decide on an impossible score (for our data set) as the line between classes.

Look at the data. Units of measure are whole numbers. It was not possible to obtain a score of 9.5. We then place our boundaries one half unit above and below the class limits for each class. This provides a clear line of demarcation between our classes. If a score is 12, since it is above 11.5 and below 13.5, we know exactly in which class to place the score. Notice that since numbers are continuous, the top boundary of one class is the same as the lower boundary of the next. Thus, we are sure to account for all of our scores—nothing falls through the cracks.

In some cases our classes will be quite wide, encompassing many scores. In such cases it becomes unwieldy to talk about a class by referring to its limits. Therefore, a shorthand way of referring to classes has been devised that permits us to use a single, representative score. The most "typical" score would be the mid-point of the class (which is equidistant from the ends of the distribution). We call this the class mark and obtain the value in one of two ways (both give you the same answer). We add either the class limits or the class boundaries together for a class then divide by two. This will often provide you with another "impossible" score. Don't worry, since this score is descriptive it's perfectly all right.

Up until now we have concentrated on the distribution of scores and ignored the frequency aspect. Now that we have established classes, we count the scores that belong in each class and enter the number under the column labeled f. Once scores have been combined into classes, we have lost information. Once I know there are three scores between 8 and 9, I no longer know which scores were 8s and which were 9s. (This is the trade-off we make when we summarize.) Always total the frequency column as a check. If you have accounted for all the scores, the sum of the numbers in the column will be the same as the number of scores you started with.

There are two other ways of looking at frequency. In cumulative frequency (*cum f*) we're interested in how many scores fall below a particular point in our distribution. Start at the lowest class and maintain a running tally of the scores. The cumulative frequency for the first class will equal the frequency for the class—there aren't any scores below the bottom of the distribution. The cumulative frequency for the next class is equal to the sum of the frequencies of the two classes. Each time you add in another class (move up a class), you simply add in the frequency of the additional class to the previous value of the cumulative frequency. When you reach the last class you're asking how many scores fall below the highest score in your data set. All of them! Thus the cumulative frequency for the highest class should equal your total number of scores.

Relative frequency (*rel f*) tells you what proportion of the total number of scores falls in a particular class. Each relative frequency will be a decimal fraction and the sum of the relative frequencies for all the classes will be 1.00 (or thereabouts, depending upon rounding error). For each class, the relative frequency is obtained by dividing the frequency for the class by the total number of scores.

Having completed our frequency distribution for our original data set, we can see the information is more orderly and easier to understand on inspection. A large data set can be summarized into a more usable form. Remember, however, that whenever we summarize we lose specific information on scores. We construct a frequency distribution when the increase in clarity outweighs this loss of specificity.

Although our space problem has been improved through the use of a frequency distribution, it would be useful if we could further distill and summarize our data. Here the mathematicians come to our aid by providing two types of scores that we can calculate to summarize our data.

□ CENTRAL TENDENCY □

For the first measure to describe our data, we want some way of describing the midpoint or "average" value in those data. Since we'll be losing some information by using a single value to represent a number of scores, we want to be sure to use the most representative value that we can obtain.

You've encountered the word "average" before. But it probably was not used in quotation marks. We're using quotes to indicate a problem with this word. "Average" is an imprecise term. We have three measures of central tendency, all calculated differently, and all can correctly be called the "average." This potential confusion is used to great advantage by those who want to lie with statistics. By reporting an "average" figure but not identifying the measure used, it is easy to mislead.

The Mean

The measure you have always called the "average" is known as the mean. We calculate a value for the mean by summing all the scores in our data and dividing by the number of scores. Since we identify scores as X values, we symbolize the mean as $\overline{X}$ and refer to it as "X bar." (If we symbolize scores with another letter, such as Y, the symbol for the mean becomes $\overline{Y}$.) To calculate the mean, we must have interval or ratio data. The formal equation for this calculation is:

$$\overline{X} = \frac{\Sigma X}{N}$$

The mean is the most useful and most commonly encountered measure of central tendency. There are three major reasons for this. First, the mean represents the midpoint or balance point of the distribution. We can measure the distance, or deviation, of each score from the mean. If we symbolize our scores as X, we refer to our measured distances as deviation scores and symbolize them with a lower case, italicized x. The sum of these deviation scores is zero for every distribution. In Table 10.2 a deviation score is calculated for each score and summed for each sample. The sum of negative scores equals the sum of the positive scores in each case. Thus the mean is the most representative value of the distributions.

In Table 10.2, the three distributions of five scores each are identical for four of the five scores. Changing one value alters the value of the mean. Therefore, the second useful characteristic of the mean is its sensitivity to all scores in a distribution. By using the mean we minimize the loss of information.

The third and final useful quality of the mean is the fact that if we draw several samples from a population and calculate their means, the mean is the most stable measure of central tendency—it will vary the least across the samples.

The Median

The second major measure of central tendency is the median. It also is second in utility value. The median is the point in a distribution of scores at which 50 percent of the scores fall above and 50 percent fall below. The actual value of the scores doesn't matter. If we have an uneven number of scores we find the median by arranging the scores in an array from lowest value to highest value and then finding the score in the middle of the array. For an even number of scores we also begin by placing the measures

TABLE 10-2 COMPARISON OF THE MEAN AND MEDIAN

Sample 1		Sample 2		Sample 3	
Raw Score	Deviation Score	Raw Score	Deviation Score	Raw Score	Deviation Score
1	−4	1	−12	1	−22
3	−2	3	−10	3	−20
4	−1	4	− 9	4	−19
7	+2	7	− 6	7	−16
10	+5	50	+37	100	+77
25	0	65	0	115	0
Mean = 5		Mean = 13		Mean = 23	
Median = 4		Median = 4		Median = 4	

in an array. Now, however, we don't have a middle score. So we go to the two middle scores and take a mean (find an average) by adding the scores and dividing by two.

The median is less sensitive to extreme scores than the mean. In Table 10.2, although the means of the three samples differ, the median value for all three samples is the same—4. In using the median rather than the mean as our measure of central tendency, we lose information. As if this weren't bad enough, the median is also less stable across samples than the mean.

The Mode

The least commonly used measure of central tendency is the mode. The mode is simply the most commonly occurring score. Table 10.3 illustrates the major weakness of the mode as a primary measure of central tendency. In Sample 1, there is no most frequent score. In Sample 2, since the score 1 occurs twice, our mode is 1. In Sample 3, both 1 and 7 occur twice. So we have two modes. That's the problem: We may have several modes, or we may have none at all. The mode is insensitive to the values of the scores in the distribution and is the least stable of the measures of central tendency.

Earlier it was mentioned that the use of the word "average" could be misleading. Suppose you were told the "average" age of patients receiving physical therapy at Nicetown Hospital was 65 years old.

Are we talking about the mean? Isn't that the first measure to come to mind? Remember, though, the mean is the balance point of the distribution. That is, the sum of the deviations below the mean must equal the sum of the deviations above it. In this case it would mean that for every patient 10 years old (55 years below the mean) we would have one patient 55 years older than the mean (120 years old!), 55 patients 66 years old, or some combination in between. So our "average" is probably not the mean.

How about the median? Is it likely that half of our patients are older

TABLE 10-3 THE MODE

Sample 1	Sample 2	Sample 3
1	1	1
3	1	1
4	4	4
7	7	7
10	10	7
No mode	One mode (Unimodal)	Two modes (Bimodal)

than 65? If the median is being used, a patient 10 years old is balanced by a patient 66 years old. All that matters is on which side of the median the patient's age falls. It's possible our average is the median, but given the number of patients younger than 65, unlikely.

So we're left with the mode. Is it conceivable that we have more patients aged 65 than any other age? Certainly.

The next time you hear about the "average" income in America, or the "average" life of a product in an advertisement, stop and think.

□ VARIABILITY □

Once we have a measure of central tendency, we have some information about the middle of the distribution. If your class "averages" 85% on your first exam and 62% on the second, you have an idea of how these compare.

However, there are several ways to arrive at the same "average." The class could average 85% with scores ranging between 70 and 100. Or, everyone in the class could receive an 85%. So we really need another measure in addition to the measure of central tendency—a measure of the spread, or variability, of scores.

The Range

The simplest form of such a measure would be to find the distance from the lowest score to the highest score in an array. This is referred to as the range. You've heard that term before in this chapter. Here we are using it in a slightly different manner. Whereas before we were counting things that happened to be numerical scores, here we really are interested in the distance between scores, not in the number of scores. So we do not add 1. To find the ranges for the classes referred to above, the range for Class One is $100 - 70 = 30$. For the second class (where everyone scored the same) the range is 0 $(85 - 85)$.

The range is a very crude measure of spread. It tells us nothing about the way scores are arranged over the span. For example, the range would be the same for the following two distributions: 1, 2, 3, 4, 100; and 1, 97, 98, 99, 100. But the distributions are very different.

Standard Deviation

Another approach would be to try to find some "average" distance of scores in the distribution from the mean. Such a score would be small for a narrow distribution (where scores were all relatively close to the mean) and large for a distribution with a great deal of spread.

In attempting to construct such a measure we almost immediately run into problems. Basically what has been proposed is finding the "average" or mean of the deviation scores. The first step in obtaining a mean is to sum all the scores. By definition, summing deviation scores results in 0.

There are several ways the problem could be evaded. The most sound mathematical method involves squaring the deviation scores. Then they can be added and divided by the number of scores. A final step would be to return to the original units of measure by taking the square root. This is essentially what we do to obtain the most commonly used measure of variability—the standard deviation. The formula is:

$$s = \sqrt{\frac{\Sigma(X - \overline{X})^2}{n - 1}}$$

Where s = standard deviation
Σ = sum
X = raw score
$\overline{X}$ = mean of distribution
n = number of measures in distribution

But wait, why are we dividing by $n - 1$ rather than the total number of measures? To understand this we must introduce a concept known as degrees of freedom. The number of degrees of freedom in a statistic tells you the number of measures that are free to vary. This implies that other measures will not be free to vary, but will be determined (can only have one value).

In calculating the mean, all measures are free to vary. (We symbolize this by: df = N.) If I know I have three measures, and I know that one is a 4, and one is a 7, there are no constraints on the value of the last number. It could be anything.

In calculating the standard deviation, we are using deviation scores. If I have an array of scores and calculate their related deviation scores, I know, by definition that these scores must sum to zero. So all but one of the scores is free to vary. When I reach that last score in my addition, the score must be one that results in a sum of zero. So for the standard deviation, the degrees of freedom (df) is equal to $n - 1$. This formula is specific to the situation where we are dealing with sample data.

The formula for s above is called the conceptual formula. By reading the formula you can understand the steps you go through to solve the problem. However, when you want to actually calculate a standard deviation you should not use this formula. For that purpose we have a computational formula that allows us to go back to the raw data and not depend on any intermediate calculations (in this case the mean). One of the corollaries of Murphy's Law is that the more calculations you perform the higher your odds of making a dumb arithmetic error. So to actually calculate a standard deviation, use the following formula:

$$s = \sqrt{\frac{\Sigma X^2 - \frac{(\Sigma X)^2}{n}}{n-1}}$$

Where X = a raw score
ΣX^2 = each raw score squared then added together
$(\Sigma X)^2$ = all the raw scores summed then the total squared

The Variance

If we eliminate the last step of the standard deviation formula (taking the square root) we have another measure of spread, known as the variance. This measure is most commonly used in the statistical technique known as Analysis of Variance (covered in this text in Chapter 12). This measure does not have much intuitive meaning since it isn't expressed in terms of the original units of measure (remember, we haven't taken the square root). So we're talking about such measures as the number of days of hospitalization squared.

Once you have calculated the mean and standard deviation of a data set you have a brief description of your distribution. These two measures are the most commonly calculated and reported measures in the research literature. For this reason we have gone into more statistical detail than we will in later sections of this text, since this is not a statistics text. In the following chapters we will concentrate on the appropriate use of the various statistical procedures, and spend less time on calculations.

□ SUMMARY □

Descriptive statistics provide a useful means for summarizing and communicating research results. Such summaries may be represented in tabular form as frequency distributions, which summarize data ranges into classes of data and describe the frequency of data within the various classes.

Data may also be described by calculated statistics that describe central tendency and variability. Measures of central tendency are the mean (the measure generally referred to by the term "average"); the median, or score that represents the point in the data array above and below which 50% of the data lie; and the mode, or most frequent score. Variability ("spread") can be described by the range, the variance, and the most frequently employed measure, the standard deviation.

□ KEY TERMS □

array	median
class mark	mode
class boundaries	deviation scores
relative frequency	variance
cumulative frequency	standard deviation
central tendency	range
mean	degrees of freedom

□□ 11 □□

Inferential Statistics: Underlying Logic

In the chapters on the various research designs we spoke repeatedly of treatment effects and interpreting evidence that would allow us to claim treatment effectiveness. The claim of treatment effectiveness is based on obtaining what we refer to as statistical significance with our results. Whereas in Chapter 10 we discussed the use of descriptive statistics to characterize and communicate our data, in Chapters 11 through 13 we will examine the various statistical techniques employed in inferential statistics.

Inferential statistics (as the name implies) involves making decisions about research results on the basis of statistical evidence. We use this evidence to draw conclusions about whether our results exhibit a strong enough effect to warrant rejecting the null hypothesis.

□ HYPOTHESIS TESTING □

To refresh your memory from Chapter 3, each research study for which statistical analysis procedures are employed consists of at least two hypotheses. The first hypothesis to be formulated when designing the study

148

is the null hypothesis (H_o). The null hypothesis is a statistical hypothesis that we test directly. It states that there was no effect for our experimental treatment or that our groups really were the same despite any apparent differences in scores. The testing of the null hypothesis is based on the laws of probability. Mathematical statisticians have calculated, for each statistical procedure, the probability of obtaining a particular value for the statistic when in fact no effect exists.

As you will recall from the example in Chapter 3 involving the coin toss, if an event is highly likely to occur by chance (for example obtaining heads when tossing a coin) and the event occurs, we are not impressed with someone's claim of having controlled the event telepathically. If we toss the coin ten times and heads appear every time (and it's a fair coin), then our skepticism toward telepathy may well begin to erode, as this outcome (ten consecutive heads) is extremely unlikely to occur by chance. It can happen—and it will, on average once in 1,000 times when a coin is tossed ten times in a row. But (again, on average) only once. Much more often we will obtain some mixture of heads and tails.

So the unlikely can occur. Maybe we have just happened on the one occasion where we would obtain our results by chance. How do we know if we really have an effect? The answer is that we never do. We can never know the true reason for obtaining our results, so statisticians have developed a set of rules governing when we reject the null hypothesis (i.e., claim that chance is not the explanation for our results).

Alpha Level

The decision on whether to reject the null hypothesis is based on the strength of the evidence—the likelihood of the results having occurred by chance. Before we begin our study we make a decision about how strong the evidence must be by establishing a cut-off or criterion point we call the alpha level (α). If we set our alpha level at .05, we are saying that we will accept the risk that five times out of 100 replications of our study the observed results would show up in the absence of an effect.

The setting of the alpha level is an arbitrary act. We can set the alpha level at .05, or if we demand stronger evidence we can set the alpha level at .01. Once set, the rules of the statistical game state that we cannot relax our standards and lower (make larger) our alpha level (e.g., go from .01 to .05). Why would we want to do this? The temptation is based on the way the alpha level is employed.

If we complete a study with an alpha level of .05, calculate a *t* test on the results, and discover that the obtained value of *t* has a probability of .03, we rejoice. The probability associated with our statistic must be as small as or smaller than our alpha level. Thus if the probability of our *t* was .05 we could still claim statistical significance and reject the null hypothesis. And we can take credit for the effect by accepting our second hypothesis—the experimental or alternative hypothesis (H_a).

To point out the arbitrariness of this game, however, let's say we conducted exactly the same experiment as above and obtained exactly the same results. That is, the probability associated with our t test value was .03. But, this time we had set our alpha level at .01. We would need a probability smaller than .01 to allow us to reject the null hypothesis. For this study, then, we would fail to reject the null hypothesis. Remember that failing to reject the null hypothesis does not mean that we are saying there is no effect. We are saying that it is one of the possible explanations for our results. Others could be poor experimental design or the use of a statistical technique that is not powerful enough to detect the effect. Given that most journals will not publish negative findings (failure to reject), can you see where the experimenter in the second study might be sorely tempted to claim the alpha level had been set at .05 all along? Is it legitimate to do this? No. Is it done? Frequently.

The alternative or experimental hypothesis is the explanation for our results that claims that the treatment is effective. As illustrated above, this hypothesis is never evaluated directly, because it is not within our power to calculate the likelihood of effects if they really exist. The statistical inference process is a probabilistic decision. Because we always state the null and experimental hypotheses so that they are mutually exclusive and exhaust the possible outcomes, the ability to reject the null hypothesis allows us to accept the alternative hypothesis.

The Decision Process

How do we know if we've drawn the correct conclusions about our experimental results? We don't. Because we never know the state of reality, the best we can try to do is to minimize our chances of being incorrect. Given that there are two considerations in the process—the state of reality and the conclusions we draw, there are two possible ways for us to be wrong.

		Conclusion Drawn	
		H_0 may be true. (Fail to reject.) (No effect appears.)	H_0 is false. (Reject null.) (Effect appears.)
State of Reality	H_0 is true (No effect)	1. Correct! Probability $= 1 - \alpha$	2. Wrong. False alarm. Type I error. Probability $= \alpha$
	H_0 is false. (Reject null)	3. Wrong. Miss. Type II error. Probability $= \beta$	4. Correct! Probability = Power or $1 - \beta$

As illustrated above, if there are two possible states of reality (always unknown to us)—that an effect does or does not exist, and two possible decisions—to reject or fail to reject the null hypothesis—we are led to four cells in a matrix combining the factors. (Please note the discrepancy in labeling in the figure.) In reality there is or is not an effect. Our possible conclusions are that there is an effect (we reject the null hypothesis) or there may not be an effect (we fail to reject). The null hypothesis admits the existence of other possible causes for our results.

Quadrants 1 and 2 demonstrate the case in which in reality an effect does not exist. In Quadrant 1 we have made a correct decision. Our conclusion to fail to reject the null hypothesis matches the real state of the universe. In Quadrant 2 we are wrong. We have chosen to conclude that an effect does exist (we reject the null hypothesis) when there is no effect. The fact is that our statistical results represented one of those times when the unlikely does occur by chance. Think of this as a false alarm (we say there is an effect and there isn't). The probability associated with making this error is within our control. It is represented by our alpha level. If we set our alpha level at .05, five times out of 100 these results will appear by chance and we'll draw the wrong conclusion. If we want to play it safer and set our alpha level at .01, only one time out of 100 will these results appear when there really is no effect. The probability of being correct and ending up on Quadrant 1 when there is no effect can be calculated by subtracting the alpha level from 1. If there is no effect and I draw the incorrect conclusion 5% of the time (alpha at .05), then I'll be correct the rest of the time (100% − 5% = 95% or .95). The error associated with Quadrant 2 has been labelled a Type I error. It is considered a potentially very serious problem, which is why we directly control the probability of making such an error.

Quadrants 3 and 4 of the figure shown above are associated with a state of reality in which our experimental treatment actually does have an effect. In this case we should reject the null hypothesis. However, in Quadrant 3 we fail to reject the null hypothesis. In other words, we fail to recognize an existing effect. We miss seeing it. This second type of error has been labeled a Type II error. The probability of making a Type II error is known as beta (β). The determination of a numerical value for beta is beyond the scope of this text.

Our final quadrant, number 4, is the happy coincidence of our recognizing an effect that does exist. The probability of being correct when an effect exists is $1 - \beta$ (through the same logic presented above). This quantity—the probability of correctly recognizing an effect—is known as power.

Just as we would rather be correct by finding an existing effect than by correctly recognizing the nonexistence of an effect, so, too, we differentially value the severity of Type I and Type II errors in the research process.

Perhaps you had an indication of this when you read that we are concerned enough about the Type I error to exercise direct control over its occurrence. In fact, Type I errors are generally considered to be more severe than Type II errors. The explanation for this may rest in the effects these errors may have on the research process.

If a Type II error is made, the researcher fails to reject the false null hypothesis. Recall that only one of the possible reasons for effects not showing up depends on the nonexistence of the effect. One possible reason we might fail to see results is that the power of either our design or our statistical technique was too low. Given that there are a number of plausible explanations for the apparent lack of an effect, a Type II error usually results in a researcher replicating the study with modifications to increase the power. In other words, the search goes on.

A Type I error, on the other hand, may result in the researcher moving on to another research problem. After all, the effect that was the basis of the research has apparently been discovered. The search is over, or it would be if an error had not been committed. In fact, the researcher believes that the effects have been found that don't really exist except as a statistical artifact. The search should continue. For this reason, researchers focus more attention and heap more abuse on the Type I error.

The probabilities associated with alpha and beta are related to each other in an indirect manner. If the researcher wants to minimize the chances of making a Type I error, the alpha level is made more stringent. The evidence must be stronger before the researcher accepts the apparent effect. By making this demand for stronger evidence, however, the researcher has increased the chances of overlooking an effect. This means that as the probability of making a Type I error is reduced, the probability of making a Type II error is increased.

□ POWER □

One way of reducing the probability of making a Type II error is to increase the power of the study. This can be done either by increasing the power of the design of the study itself or by increasing the power of the statistical methods employed. Any changes in the design that enhance the probability of noticing an effect increase power. The most common ways of increasing design power involve: (1) increasing the potency of the independent variable manipulation, (2) reducing noise in the study, (3) increasing the number of subjects employed, and (4) using a less stringent alpha level (e.g., .05 instead of .01).

Increasing the potency of the independent variable is likely to increase the size of the effect. Larger experimental effects are easier to see. One option open to the researcher is to employ several levels of the independent variable manipulation with at least one being large (or powerful) enough to virtually ensure recognition of effects.

Noise in the study can be reduced by adopting procedures that decrease the irrelevant variability in the measures. One method may be to introduce a repeated measures design in which subjects serve as their own controls. As mentioned previously, this technique greatly reduces within-subject variability—in a pre- to post-test design the researcher is assured that the subject is, except for the experimental treatment, essentially the same in terms of nuisance characteristics that might influence scores on the dependent variable.

Increasing the number of subjects in the study works both at the design and the statistical levels to increase power. Employing more sources of data is a design consideration. However, most statistical tests are evaluated in terms of the probabilities associated with specific outcomes on the number of degrees of freedom in the design (see Chapter 11). In most cases the number of degrees of freedom is at least indirectly associated with the number of subjects in the study. The rule of thumb is that the larger the *n* (number of subjects) the smaller an effect need be to achieve statistical significance.

□ ILLUSTRATION OF STATISTICAL INFERENCE □

At this point your head may be spinning with all of these unfamiliar concepts and terms. Let's go back to the beginning and concretize the ideas through an admittedly silly example.

It's summer vacation and I'm going to enjoy the beauties of nature by going off into the woods camping alone. My friends warn me about the bears in the woods, but I ignore their advice and set out on my merry way.

About a hundred yards short of the creek where I intend to camp I pass an encampment of Boy Scouts, who mark my passing with such pleasantries as "Hey, lady, the bears are going to get you!" and giggles. I, of course, ignore them.

I reach my campsite, set up camp, eat dinner, and zip myself into my tent to sleep. I'm awakened by a noise in the campsite. Is it a bear? I'm not about to look outside to find out.

OK. My null hypothesis is that the state of reality is that there's no bear out there. I'm imagining things, it's the wind, or some small animal. My alternative or experimental hypothesis is that there is too a bear out there. So my decision matrix becomes:

| | **My Conclusion** | |
	No bear. (Fail to reject.) (H_0 may be true)	Bear!!! (Reject null.) (H_0 is false)
Reality No bear	1. Correct	2. Wrong. False alarm. Type I error.
Bear!!!	3. Wrong! Miss. Type II error.	4. Correct

How will I decide which conclusion to draw? I collect evidence. I listen.
I've decided that if I conclude there is a bear I'm swallowing my pride and
racing down to the Boy Scouts. So the evidence better be pretty convincing. In other words, I'm setting my alpha level so it is unlikely I'll decide
there's a bear if there isn't one.

Let's first look at the case in which there is no bear in my campsite (H_o
is true). I might decide after listening that there isn't a bear and go back to
sleep. I'd be in Quadrant 1 and I'd be correct. Or, I could listen, decide
there's enough evidence to convince me, and run screaming down the
trail. I come back with the snickering scouts and (oops) a skunk has got-
ten into my trash. False alarm.

Or it could be that there is a bear outside my tent. The bear might be
very quiet and I might decide I don't have a reason to believe it's out there
(the sounds I'm hearing might easily be made by some small, harmless animal) and I go back to sleep. Until I am joined in my tent by the bear. Finally, I can decide there is a bear when there certainly is one and escape to
safety with no loss of face.

In this example my Type I error is crying wolf (or in this case, bear). It's
a false alarm. There isn't a bear. My Type II error is missing the presence of
a very real effect. The power of the study is my ability to make a correct
decision about the presence of the bear. (Please note that in this example
there may be some question as to which type of error is more severe. To
the extent that academicians might prefer bodily injury to loss of dignity,
the example holds up.)

□ EVALUATING RESULTS □

A statistic is a number. We conduct an *F* test, or a *t* test, or an *H* test and
our result is a number. For most statistical procedures this number has no
inherent meaning. It must be evaluated as to the probability of obtaining
this value for the statistic if the null hypothesis is true. Fortunately for us,
our friends the mathematical statisticians have calculated these probabilities and publish tables that allow us to evaluate our research results.
These tables are based on probability distributions and allow us to determine whether our obtained statistic falls within the region of rejection.
The region of rejection is that portion of the distribution that contains
scores for the statistic that allow us to reject the null hypothesis. If our alpha level is .05, then 5% of the area of the distribution will be in the region
of rejection. We take the number we have obtained through our calculations and compare it to the "critical value" of the statistic obtained from
the appropriate table. For most statistical tables, if our obtained value is as
large as, or larger than, the critical value we assume that our effect or
group difference is large enough to allow us to reject the null hypothesis.

□ SUMMARY □

Hypothesis testing is the process of employing the research data to evaluate the research hypotheses. Evidence (data) has been collected that will allow the researcher to evaluate the probability that the null hypothesis is false. If the researcher is able to reject the null hypothesis, the alternative or experimental hypothesis is accepted.

Before beginning to collect data, the investigator defines the level of evidence that will be considered as strong enough to enable rejection of the null hypothesis. This criterion level is known as the alpha level. Incorrect rejection of the null hypothesis is known as a Type I error and is considered extremely serious; therefore, an alpha level of at least .05 is usually employed. If the probability that the obtained value for the statistic is the result of chance is as low as or lower than our alpha level, we say the statistic falls within the region of rejection, we reject the null hypothesis, and accept the experimental hypothesis.

The alternative error, failing to recognize an effect that does exist, is known as a Type II error. Power is defined as the ability to detect an existing effect.

□ KEY TERMS □

alpha level
beta
power
type I error

type II error
region of rejection
critical value

□□ 12 □□

Inferential Statistics for Pre-Experimental and True Experimental Research

□ *Parametric Tests*
  □ *t Tests*
  □ *Analysis of Variance*
  □ *Analysis of Covariance*
□ *Nonparametric Tests*
  □ *Wilcoxon Signed Rank Test*
  □ *Wilcoxon Rank Sum Test*
  □ *Kruskal-Wallis Test*

This is not a statistics textbook. Therefore, the following descriptions of statistical techniques will remain primarily at the conceptual level. For some of the less complex techniques, formulas will be presented. The more complex calculations will be presented in the Appendix at the end of the chapter. Recognizing the prevalence of math and statistics phobias, let us hasten to point out that it is possible to at least begin to grasp this material by reading only the text the first time through. Once the concepts are firmly at your command you will recognize that equations merely represent diagrams or road maps of how to calculate a statistic from the starting point of raw data.

□ PARAMETRIC TESTS □

The first group of statistical techniques we will explore is made up of the *parametric tests*. This label refers to the fact that certain underlying assumptions, or parameters, must be met (the data must possess certain characteristics) before these techniques may be employed.

The first of these assumptions is that the sampling distributions of the variables possess a normal shape. (The normal distribution is discussed in Chapter 15). Briefly, the normal curve is a bell-shaped, symmetrical distribution for which the mean, median, and mode all fall at the midpoint of the range. The normal distribution possesses some very handy mathematical characteristics, which have been used in the development of the parametric tests.

The second assumption is that the variances of the variable distributions must be equivalent. This is known as homogeneity of variance. All this essentially means is that if the scores are spread out for one variable (i.e., the variance is large), they must have a similar dispersion for any comparison variable.

Parametric tests are quite powerful—much more so than their counterparts, the nonparametric tests. Fortunately, they are also robust. This means that the underlying assumptions can be violated to a moderate degree without the integrity of the tests being destroyed. Since a powerful test is more likely to recognize existing effects, the use of parametric tests is highly desirable.

t *Tests*

The *t* tests are a set of techniques developed by Gosset under the pseudonym "Student." The three tests apply to three research designs. All of the tests compare the means of two groups (e.g., a pre- and a post-treatment score). For all three the larger the discrepancy between the scores, the larger the obtained value for *t* and the greater the likelihood that the *t* value will fall in the region of rejection, allowing rejection of the null hypothesis. For all three tests the null hypothesis states that the means of the two groups being compared are equal. The three tests are (1) the single sample *t*, (2) the correlated groups *t*, and (3) the independent groups *t*.

Single Sample t *Test*   The single sample *t* test compares the mean for a sample against the population mean for a particular variable. You will recall that we seldom have access to population data. For this reason this test is not all that commonly encountered. For some characteristics, however, we either have access to population data, or we have data on such very large samples that for all practical purposes they can be considered population data.

For example, although not everyone in the United States has been given a standardized IQ test, enough such tests have been administered over a long enough period that behavioral scientists accept the range of 90–110 as the "average" IQ (a mean of 100 and a standard deviation of 16 for the Stanford Binet test).

We might employ this test, then, if we had reason to believe (as some do) that IQ is a question of nurture or training and we wanted to test the effectiveness of a technique we believed would increase IQ in our treatment group. We would randomly choose a sample of subjects, administer our treatment, and measure the IQ of subjects post-treatment. (Notice the lack of a pretest.)

In our present example we predicted that the treatment would increase IQ. This is called a directional hypothesis. Our prediction is that $X - \mu > 0$. This will result in a positive value for t. Thus our region of rejection will lie at the positive end of the t distribution. If our alpha level is .05, our region of rejection (shaded in Fig. 12-1) will begin with the score (value of t) that divides off the top 5% of the area of the distribution. (The values along the horizontal axis are values of t scores.) Thus the name *one-tailed test*. The obtained t must be positive in sign and as large as or larger than the critical value for significance.

Suppose we expected our treatment to change IQ but we were unwilling to predict the direction of the change. We would be equally interested in $X - \mu > 0$ and in $X - \mu < 0$. The only case that would cause us to fail to reject the null hypothesis would be $X - \mu = 0$. A hypothesis of this kind is called a nondirectional hypothesis.

With a nondirectional distribution, we have to consider a region of rejection at both ends of the distribution. However, if we retain our alpha level at .05 we must still include in our region of rejection 5% of the distribution. Thus we cut off 2.5% at each end of the distribution, as seen in Figure 12-2.

For the example we have been following, using 49 degrees of freedom (our n was 50), the critical value for a one-tailed t test would be $+1.645$. For a two-tailed t test, the critical value would be ± 1.960. In either event our obtained value of 11.7848 would allow us to reject the null hypothesis.

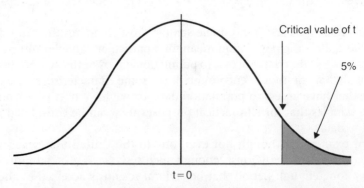

Critical value of t

5%

t = 0

FIGURE 12-1   Region of rejection for a directional hypothesis (one-tailed) with an alpha level of .05.

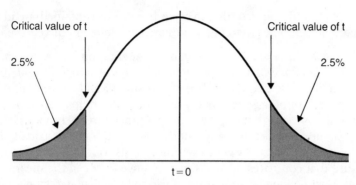

FIGURE 12-2 *Region of rejection for a non-directional hypothesis (two-tailed test) with an alpha level of .05.*

Let us say, however, that we had predicted our treatment would increase IQ and we found instead the mean sample IQ after treatment had dropped to 80? Our obtained value of t would be -11.7848. Since we made a directional prediction we use a one-way test just as in the initial condition: we need a value of $+1.645$ or greater in order to reject the null hypothesis. In this case we must fail to reject the null hypothesis. As you can see, it is important to be careful in choosing whether to employ a directional or nondirectional experimental hypothesis. This decision is not necessary in all cases. The probability distributions associated with some statistical techniques (such as the chi square) allow only for one-tailed tests.

Correlated Groups t *Test*   The correlated groups t test is employed when we have the subjects as their own control group. For each subject, then, we have a pretreatment and a post-treatment score. The null hypothesis says the treatment was not effective—that is, that all differences between pretreatment and post-treatment scores are zero.

The basic idea of this test is analogous to that of the single sample test discussed above. The size of the mean difference between pretreatment and post-treatment is divided by a measure of dispersion of the difference scores. The results of this t test are evaluated as described above.

The correlated groups t test is also employed when groups consist of separate individuals who have been matched on some characteristic. Matching is used to control for a variable that, while not of interest in the particular study, might affect the dependent variable. For example, if the dependent variable is the number of days it takes stroke victims to recover enough mobility to take ten unaided steps, differences in patient age might confound any differences between treatments. Thus we would match the treatment groups by age—for each very old patient in one group, we would be sure that every other group contained a patient of comparable age. The difference scores are calculated on matched pairs.

Independent Groups t *Test*   In the independent groups *t* test we compare the means obtained on our dependent measures by two independent samples. Usually these two groups are our treatment and control groups. We do not match or otherwise actively seek to create comparable groups. The assumption is made that the use of proper procedures of random selection and assignment will cause any interfering variables to be equally represented in our groups. As with the other *t* tests, our statistic consists of a measure that compares means (the difference between the means of our two groups) divided by a measure of variability calculated by pooling the variability in our two groups.

Analysis of Variance (ANOVA)

The major disadvantage of the *t* tests is that they allow us to compare only two groups at a time. Suppose, as in the nonequivalent control group design with separate pre- and post-test samples, we wish to compare more than two groups? We could in theory just perform multiple *t* tests. In practice this would not be a sound idea. When we set an alpha level we establish the probability of a Type I error for that test alone. When we perform multiple *t* tests we lose control of the alpha level and suffer an increased probability of a Type I error.

$$
\begin{array}{cccl}
0 & | & 0 & \text{Group 1 (control)} \\
  & | & & \\
0 & | \ X & 0 & \text{Group 2 (treatment)}
\end{array}
$$

For the design above, let us label the observation points as follows: A = Control pretest, B = Control post-test, C = Treatment pretest, and D = Treatment post-test. In order to make the desired comparisons we would have to perform six separate *t* tests.

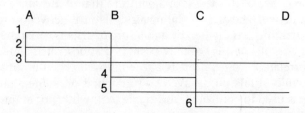

The analysis of variance (ANOVA) tests allow us to make all of these comparisons at one time while maintaining the desired alpha level. The statistic calculated is the *F*, which is evaluated using standardized tables.

The major variations of the ANOVA are the one-way ANOVA, which tests multiple levels (2 +) of one independent variable on the dependent measure(s); the factorial ANOVA, which assesses the effects of multiple levels of more than one independent variable; and the repeated-measures ANOVA, which measures the dependent variable(s) on more than one occasion. The ANOVA tests are parametric tests.

When we calculate a value for F we have the advantage of knowing that our alpha level has remained under control despite the number of comparisons made. The disadvantage is that if, for example, in the design above our F fell in the region of rejection we could reject the null hypothesis and claim that at least one of the comparisons was significantly larger than we would expect to see by chance. However, at this point we could not say which comparison was significant. Further tests, known as post hoc tests, must be conducted to find the significant difference(s). There are a number of different post hoc tests that make and evaluate pairwise comparisons. You will find a discussion of these tests in a statistics textbook.

$$F = \frac{\text{Between-group variance estimate}}{\text{Within-group variance estimate}}$$

Essentially the F statistic is a ratio between two variance estimates. The variability within groups (the denominator) we believe to be the naturally occurring random variability we would expect to see in any group of people. We believe that the difference between the groups has been created through our experimental treatment or intervention. An effective treatment would create larger differences between our groups than we find within our groups. Generally an F of one or less is not worth evaluating. A negative value of F indicates that computations have gone awry, since it is possible to have no variation (represented by a value of zero) but it is not possible to have less than no variation.

The factorial analysis of variance, as mentioned above, examines the effects of multiple levels of more than one independent variable on the dependent measures of interest. In addition to providing information about the effects of each independent variable separately, the factorial ANOVA provides unique information on possible interactions between the independent variables that can be obtained in no other way.

For example, let us consider a study that examines the effectiveness of two training programs designed to increase the nutritional levels of meals self-prepared by elderly individuals. Type of program would be one independent variable with two levels, in-home individual training or group classes at a community facility. The second independent variable could be gender of the client. The dependent measure would be the nutritional level of meals prepared by clients.

		Programs	
		A	B
Gender	M	G1	G2
	F	G3	G4

This design would allow us to determine if one training program was more effective than the other for all clients (men and women); whether gender differences in clients alone made a difference on the dependent measure, independent of the training program; and, finally, whether male clients responded to the different training programs in the same manner as female clients. An example of an interaction effect would be the finding that male clients responded more favorably to the home training whereas the female clients responded to the group classes. Only the use of the factorial ANOVA would allow us to uncover this effect.

Analysis of Covariance (ANCOVA)

Occasionally in research (probably more often than experimenters would like to believe) nuisance variables crop up that may affect the dependent variable but are irrelevant to our independent variables. These nuisance variables may interfere with the analysis of our data by providing a source of noise that obscures the effects the research is intended to examine. The analysis of covariance is a technique that to some extent reduces the effect of these extraneous variables.

For example, consider a training program designed to accelerate increases in muscular strength in limbs that have been immobilized in casts. This training program is administered to patients of all ages. But age may represent a nuisance variable: younger patients might regain strength more quickly solely because of their youth. In this case using an analysis of covariance with age as a covariate would to some extent pull the variability associated with age out of the data. The transformed data would then be analyzed for the effect of the training program. The technique calculates a corrected score for each subject then analyzes the corrected scores using the standard analysis of variance procedures. The procedure is not foolproof, however, and may (as described in Chapter 5) overcorrect or undercorrect the data and lead to biased statistical results.

□ NONPARAMETRIC TESTS □

Nonparametric tests are not as powerful as their parametric counterparts, and they may fail to detect an effect that would be detected with a parametric test. They do not, however, rest on any underlying assumptions and should be employed when the underlying assumptions necessary for use of parametric procedures are seriously violated—for example, when the distribution is known to be non-normal in shape. Unlike the parametric tests, the nonparametric tests do not focus on the mean. The null hypothesis for the nonparametric tests considered in this chapter states that the probability distributions of the populations of the groups being compared are identical. In this chapter we consider three of the nonparametric tests, chosen because they represent the nonparametric equivalents to the parametric techniques already discussed. We will discuss the Wilcoxon signed rank test (equivalent to the corelated groups *t* test), the Wilcoxon rank sum test (equivalent to the *t* test for independent groups), and the Kruskal-Wallis test (equivalent to the one-way analysis of variance).

Wilcoxon Signed Rank Test

The Wilcoxon signed rank test is performed on data that consist of paired scores, either pre- and post-test scores on individuals or scores on matched pairs. The calculations in this test are very simple. Difference scores are obtained for each subject. Some of these difference scores will be positive in value, some will be negative. The difference scores are ranked in order of absolute value, with the smallest absolute difference receiving a rank of 1. Once all scores are ranked, the sign of the difference again becomes salient. All ranks associated with positive differences are summed, as are all ranks associated with negative differences. The smaller of these two sums is evaluated using a standardized table. The smaller the value, the greater the evidence of differences between the scores. This is one of the few cases where the obtained value for the statistic must be as small as or smaller than the critical value obtained from the table if the null hypothesis is to be rejected.

Wilcoxon Rank Sum Test

The Wilcoxon Rank Sum Test is the equivalent of the *t* test for independent groups. For this test ranks are assigned to scores on the dependent variable for all subjects in the study, with the lowest score receiving the rank of 1. Subjects are divided into their experimental groups and the ranks for each group are summed. The possible values for the sum of the ranks are constrained by the fact that the sum of all ranks in the study will always equal

$$\frac{n(n+1)}{2}$$

Thus, if the sum of ranks for Group 1 is small, the sum for Group 2 must account for the remainder of the value of this equation.

Tables used to evaluate this statistic provide two values (representing the two summed ranks). The smaller of the two ranked sums must be smaller than or equal to the smaller of the tabled values *or* the larger ranked sum must be equal to or larger than the larger of the two tabled values if the null hypothesis is to be rejected.

Kruskal-Wallis Test

The Kruskal-Wallis test is the nonparametric equivalent of the one-way analysis of variance. Like other nonparametric tests this test is based on rankings of scores on the dependent measure where all subjects are initially treated as one group (during the ranking procedure).

Calculations are often much simpler and more straighforward in nonparametric than in parametric tests. However, nonparametric tests can entail such a dramatic loss in power that they should only be employed when the researcher has reason to believe that the underlying assumptions of the parametric tests are seriously violated. As far as calculations are concerned, today almost all calculations are carried out by computer, so ease of calculation has ceased to be a major consideration.

□ SUMMARY □

Parametric tests are employed for true experimental designs when the underlying assumptions of homogeneity of variance and normal distribution of the sampling distributions are met. Parametric tests are extremely powerful tests that are fairly robust (i.e., able to withstand moderate violations of the underlying assumptions). The various *t* tests are employed for comparisons between the means of two groups. The analysis of variance allows for comparisons of the means of more than two groups while still maintaining the probability of a Type I error at the chosen alpha level. The analysis of covariance reduces the effect of extraneous variables on analysis of the dependent measures.

Nonparametric tests are employed as a fall-back when the more powerful parametric tests are inappropriate. The Wilcoxon Signed Rank Test is the equivalent of the *t* test for Single Samples and Correlated Groups, the Wilcoxon Rank Sum Test is the equivalent of the Independent Groups *t* test, and the Kruskal-Wallis Test is the nonparametric equivalent of the one-way analysis of variance.

□ KEY TERMS □

parametric tests
homogeneity of variance
t tests
single sample *t* test
correlated groups *t* test
independent groups *t* test

analysis of variance (ANOVA)
analysis of covariance (ANCOVA)
nonparametric tests
Wilcoxon signed rank test
Wilcoxon rank sum test
Kruskal-Wallis test

□ APPENDIX—CALCULATION OF *t* TESTS AND ANOVA □

The statistical procedures presented in Chapter 12 were presented only descriptively. This appendix provides the means to calculate the various *t* tests—tests that the novice researcher might actually wish to employ for a research project. Formulas for the remaining tests may be found in any standard statistics textbook.

All *t* tests share the same basic form. The actual value of *t* is calculated as a ratio between two values—a comparison of values of means divided by a measure of variability. Of course, the calculations employed to obtain these values vary depending on the particular test under consideration. For all tests a large value for *t* is desirable and more likely (when evaluated) to indicate statistical significance.

Single Sample t Test

The single sample *t* test involves comparing the mean of a single sample against a known population mean.

$$t = \frac{\overline{X} - \mu}{s/\sqrt{n}}$$

Where $\overline{X}$ = sample mean
μ = population mean
s = sample standard deviation
n = number of subjects

The mean population value for IQ is 100. Let's say the obtained mean IQ score for our sample was 120. It certainly is higher than the population mean, but is the difference large enough to be significant? If we had chosen 50 subjects, with an obtained standard deviation in scores of 12, our calculations would look like this:

$$t = \frac{120 - 100}{12/\sqrt{50}} = \frac{20}{1.6971} = 11.7848$$

Is a *t* of 11.7848 within the region of rejection? To determine this we must use a standardized table. To use the table we must have two pieces of information. First we need to calculate the number of degrees of freedom. Recall from our discussion of variability that one degree of freedom is lost in calculating the standard deviation. Since we calculated the standard deviation as part of this formula, the degrees of freedom for the single-sample *t* is $n - 1$ (the number of subjects minus one).

The second piece of information we need to evaluate our results is information on whether we are conducting a one-tailed or a two-tailed test. This determination is based on our experimental hypothesis and determines the distribution of the region of rejection.

Once we have these pieces of information we would obtain what is known as the critical value of the statistic from the table. If our obtained value is as large as or larger than the critical value we claim statistical significance.

Correlated Groups t Test

The formula used to calculate this type of *t* test has much in common with the single-sample *t* test. Since we are interested in difference scores (for each subject, obtained by subtracting the pre-treatment score from the post-treatment score, and symbolized as *D*) we again have one group of scores. The top of the formula compares the mean of the obtained difference scores to the mean of the population of difference scores if the null hypothesis is true. If the null hypothesis is true, all difference scores are zero, so this term drops out of computations. The denominator of the equation is again a measure of variability.

$$t = \frac{\overline{D} - \mu_D}{s_{\overline{D}}}$$

Where $\overline{D}$ = mean of difference scores
μ_D = mean of population of difference scores
$s_{\overline{D}}$ = standard deviation of the mean of difference scores

$s_{\overline{D}}$ is a standard deviation of the mean of the difference scores. To calculate this value, recall that the standard deviation is the square root of the variance—the variance of the mean of the difference scores. The formula for the variance is:

$$\frac{s_D^2}{n}$$

To get the standard deviation we will have to take the square root of this value. The denominator of this variance is clear enough, but what does the numerator represent? This is the variance of the difference scores (not the mean of the difference scores). The formula for this variance ($S^2{}_D$) is:

$$\frac{\Sigma(D - \overline{D})^2}{n - 1}$$

This formula is familiar. If we substitute X for D we have the formula for a sample variance as seen in Chapter 10. The numerator is known as the sum of squares and has the following computational formula:

$$\Sigma(D - \overline{D})^2 = \Sigma D^2 - \frac{(\Sigma D)^2}{n}$$

Now we can follow our trail of breadcrumbs back to the original formula as follows:

$$\Sigma(D - \overline{D})^2 = \Sigma D^2 - \frac{(\Sigma D)^2}{n}$$

$$s_D^2 = \frac{\Sigma(D - \overline{D})^2}{n - 1}$$

$$s_{\overline{D}} = \sqrt{s_{\overline{D}}^2} \longleftrightarrow s_{\overline{D}}^2 = \frac{s_D^2}{n}$$

so: $$s_{\overline{D}}^2 = \frac{\Sigma D^2 - \frac{(\Sigma D)^2}{n}}{n - 1}$$

and: $$s_{\overline{D}}^2 = \frac{\left(\dfrac{\Sigma D^2 - \dfrac{(\Sigma D)^2}{n}}{n - 1}\right)}{n} \quad \text{or} \quad \frac{\Sigma D^2 - \dfrac{(\Sigma D)^2}{n}}{n(n - 1)}$$

therefore: $$s_{\overline{D}} = \sqrt{\frac{\Sigma D^2 - \dfrac{(\Sigma D)^2}{n}}{n(n - 1)}}$$

The obtained statistic is evaluated as explained above. The number of degrees of freedom for this test is again $n - 1$, where n represents the number of pairs of scores.

Independent Groups t Test

Again, our formula consists of a numerator that compares means and a denominator that represents a measure of variability, in this case a measure that combines or pools the variability of the two samples. The additional term

$$t = \frac{\overline{X}_1 - \overline{X}_2 - \mu_{\overline{x}_1 - \overline{x}_2}}{s_D}$$

Where $\overline{X}_1$ = mean of Sample 1
$\overline{X}_2$ = mean of Sample 2
$\mu_{\overline{x}_1 - \overline{x}_2}$ = mean of population of differences between Samples 1 and 2
s_D = pooled variance of Samples 1 and 2

in the numerator ($\mu_{\overline{x}_1 - \overline{x}_2}$) represents the mean of the population of difference scores obtained by comparing means of Samples 1 and 2. If the null hypothesis is true, all such scores are zero and the term drops off the equation.

Let's employ a diagram similar to that used above to illustrate the calculation of S_D.

$$\Sigma x_1{}^2 = \Sigma X_1{}^2 - \frac{(\Sigma X_1)^2}{n_1}$$

$$\Sigma x_2{}^2 = \Sigma X_2{}^2 - \frac{(\Sigma X_2)^2}{n_2}$$

$$s_D = \sqrt{s^2 \left(\frac{1}{n_1} + \frac{1}{n_2} \right)} \qquad s^2 = \frac{\Sigma x_1{}^2 + \Sigma x_2{}^2}{n_1 + n_2 - 2}$$

So: $$s^2 = \frac{\Sigma X_1{}^2 - \dfrac{(\Sigma X_1)^2}{n_1} + \Sigma X_2{}^2 - \dfrac{(\Sigma X_2)^2}{n_2}}{n_1 + n_2 - 2}$$

and $$s_D = \sqrt{\left(\frac{\Sigma X_1{}^2 - \dfrac{(\Sigma X_1)^2}{n_1} + \Sigma X_2{}^2 - \dfrac{(\Sigma X_2)^2}{n_2}}{n_1 + n_2 - 2} \right) \left(\frac{1}{n_1} + \frac{1}{n_2} \right)}$$

The obtained value of *t* is evaluated as discussed above, however the number of degrees of freedom is $n_1 + n_2 - 2$ (where n_1 is the number of subjects in group one, and n_2 is the number of subjects in group two).

Analysis of Variance (ANOVA)

The ANOVA makes use of means in calculating the statistic. The null hypothesis is always that the means of the treatment groups are equal. Besides means for each sample group, we also use a value known as the grand mean and symbolized variously as $\overline{X}_G$ or $\overline{\overline{X}}$. The grand mean is just a mean calculated using all the subjects in the study. The measure of between-group variability represents comparisons between the mean for each group and the grand mean for the study. The within-groups (also known as within-subjects) variability estimate represents comparisons within each group of individual scores to the mean for their group.

As the calculation of the ANOVA is somewhat tedious we will not present formulas. Instead, we will trace the following schematic, which illustrates the steps involved in the calculation of an F.

$$F = \frac{\text{Between-groups variance estimate}}{\text{Within-groups variance estimate}} \nearrow \frac{\text{Sum of squares (between groups)}}{\text{df (between groups)} = k - 1}$$
$$\searrow \frac{\text{Sum of squares (within groups)}}{\text{df (within groups)} = N - k}$$

A sum of squares is calculated for each source of variability. For the one-way ANOVA this is between groups and within groups. These sums of squares are converted into the variance estimates (also known as mean squares) by dividing by the appropriate degrees of freedom. The degrees of freedom for between-group variability is calculated as $k - 1$ where k represents the number of levels of the independent variable (the number of groups). The degrees of freedom for the within-group variability estimate is calculated as $N - k$ where N is the total number of subjects in the study (the sum of all groups) and k again represents the number of groups. The obtained F is evaluated using the degrees of freedom for both the numerator and denominator of the ratio.

Inferential Statistics for Quasi-
and Non-Experimental Research

□ *Chi Square*
□ *Correlation*
    □ *Spearman Correlation*
    □ *Pearson Product-Moment Correlation*
□ *Linear Regression*
□ *Coefficient of Determination*
□ *Multiple Regression*
□ *Time Series Analysis*
□ *Interrupted Time Series Analysis*

The statistical techniques discussed in this chapter are employed for data analysis on research studies using either quasi-experimental or non-experimental designs such as those discussed in Chapters 5 and 6. Like the techniques presented in the previous chapter, these statistical procedures allow the researcher to determine (according to the rules of the statistical game presented in Chapter 11) whether to reject the null hypothesis. The first procedure we will discuss also allows the researcher to assess the equivalence of samples to the population by determining whether characteristics are distributed in the same pattern in both the sample and the population.

As in previous chapters, actual calculations are held to a minimum and formulas are presented only for the less complex techniques. More sophisticated procedures (such as time series analysis) are discussed conceptually. As will be seen in Chapter 14, most (if not all) of these analyses are routinely conducted by computers.

□ CHI SQUARE □

The chi square tests are a set of three procedures (simple chi square, contingency chi square, and goodness of fit) that allow the researcher to determine whether the actual outcome of an event matches the predicted outcome. For example, if we toss a coin twelve times and come up with two heads, how does that compare to the number of heads we could expect by chance? The primary drawback of the chi-square test is that it uses nominal data and consequently only a limited number of mathematical approaches can be used. The data used for analysis are counts of category membership (in this case "heads").

This test is useful in survey research or in any case where the researcher is concerned about the similarities between groups of subjects. If the researcher can determine the distribution of characteristics such as gender or age (or anything else the researcher feels may affect the dependent measure), then a chi-square test on the respondents will test whether the sample matches the population. This information may be particularly important in assessing whether attrition from initially equivalent groups has altered their equivalence.

The chi-square tests all employ the same two basic formulas. The first formula represents the general case of the test. The chi square statistic is evaluated using the number of degrees of freedom and a standardized table. (The degrees of freedom is determined differently for each type of chi square, as discussed below.) Whenever the degrees of freedom is more than 1, the following formula is used:

$$\chi^2 = \sum \frac{(f_o - f_e)^2}{f_e}$$
Where f_o = observed frequency
f_e = expected frequency

The calculated value obtained through this procedure is evaluated with standardized tables that list the critical values for the various degrees of freedom. When the obtained chi square value equals or exceeds the critical value, the null hypothesis is rejected.

However, when there is only one degree of freedom, employing the above formula in conjunction with standardized tables results in a distortion of the inference process. Recall that the values in the tables are based on probability distributions for the statistics. The shape of the distribution for one degree of freedom is so different that the values in the table overestimate the effect. The critical values for the tables for one degree of freedom when used in conjunction with the standard formula overestimate the size of the effect and increase the probability of a Type I error through evaluation error.

There is a way around this problem, which is fortunate since chi square problems often have only one degree of freedom. Yates has developed a corrected chi square formula that corrects the obtained figure so that the tables may be appropriately employed.

$$\chi^2 = \sum \frac{(|f_o - f_e| - .5)^2}{f_e}$$

For each group a constant of .5 is subtracted from the absolute value of the difference between the observed and expected frequencies before the quantity is squared. The figures obtained for each group are summed as before and the chi square is evaluated.

The degrees of freedom for the simple chi square and the "goodness of fit" chi square are both determined by subtracting one from the number of groups in the study ($k - 1$). Note that the number of subjects is not relevant here.

The null hypothesis for the simple chi square states that the distribution of subjects will be equal across groups. A chi square test on patients' preferences for private versus semi-private hospital rooms would test the null hypothesis that 50% of any number of subjects would choose each option — that is, that there would be no preference. If there were a third choice available (perhaps a ward), the null hypothesis would state that one third would choose each option. Since the experimental hypothesis in such a study is most usually that there is a difference, rejecting the null hypothesis is the researcher's fondest hope.

Not so for the goodness-of-fit test. For the goodness-of-fit test the researcher is hoping that the pattern of responses or characteristics is the same for the sample and the comparison group (usually the population). A large chi square here would indicate that the patterns differ significantly. This would be bad news for a researcher hoping to prove equivalence. Thus, for this type of chi square the hope is for a small value for chi square, which indicates a good fit. In that case the null hypothesis of "no difference" is not rejected.

The final type of chi square test assesses the independence of two characteristics as they influence responses. Let's discuss the simplest case where we have two independent variables. The null hypothesis states that the two variables are independent of each other. To test this we set up what is known as a contingency table.

Let's look at a study of physical therapists who have been polled about how they feel about a research design course being made a requirement in the training of physical therapists. In the sample are both male and female therapists. The null hypothesis would state that attitude toward the requirement would be independent of the gender of the therapist. The contingency table for this problem would be set up as follows:

**Gender of
Therapist**
Male   Female

		Male	Female
Attitude	For		
	Against		

Within each of the cells of the table would go the counts associated with that category (e.g. male therapists in favor of the requirement). A large value of chi square would reject the null hypothesis and state that attitude is contingent (dependent) on therapist gender.

The degrees of freedom for a contingency chi square is calculated as $(r - 1)(c - 1)$ where r = the number of rows in the table and c = the number of columns in the table. In this example we have one degree of freedom, so the Yates' corrected formula should be employed.

For the contingency chi square the calculation of expected frequencies is the most challenging part of the analysis. Basically, expected frequencies are calculated on the basis of the proportions appearing in the sample — based on the assumption that the null hypothesis is true. (If that makes no sense, don't panic. If you need it, look it up in any statistics text for a more comprehensive explanation.)

□ CORRELATION □

Whenever variables are measured but not manipulated the researcher is only able to determine the extent to which variation within a pair of variables is similar. As has been mentioned, the statistics that measure this covariation are known as correlations. There are a number of different correlation coefficients whose use depends on the form of the data to be analyzed. We will discuss only two: the Spearman and the Pearson correlation coefficients.

Correlation coefficients are unusual in the world of statistics in that the actual value of the calculated statistic has inherent meaning — often of more interest than the probability associated with the outcome. In fact, for the Pearson coefficient, the obtained value must be further transformed (into a t equivalent) to allow for determination of statistical significance.

Correctly calculated correlation coefficients vary in value from -1 through 0 to $+1$. It is not possible to have a value larger than $+1$ or smaller than -1 because a coefficient of 1 represents a perfect relationship. The value of the coefficient indicates the size of the relationship, the sign indicates the direction of the relationship.

A correlation of 1 (either $+1$ or -1) indicates a perfect linear relationship between variables. This means that variation in one variable is always related to variation in the other. As the coefficient becomes smaller (closer to 0), the synchronicity between variables is reduced. A correlation of 0 indicates the total lack of a linear relationship between the variables.

If $+1$ and -1 both indicate a perfect relationship between variables, what's the difference? The sign of a correlation coefficient describes the pattern of the relationship. In a positive correlation the values of the variables change in the same direction. There is a positive correlation between human height and weight (although by no means a perfect relationship). Taller people tend to be heavier. Short people tend to be lighter.

In a negative correlation, the variables move in opposite directions. For example, air temperature is negatively correlated with the number of layers of clothing worn: As the temperature goes up, the number of layers of clothing goes down.

A calculated correlation coefficient, then, provides useful information in and of itself. In fact, many investigators dispense entirely with calculating the statistical significance of the statistic. There is also another reason not to bother to calculate the probability associated with a correlation. The transformed value is evaluated using degrees of freedom. Recall that the degrees of freedom figure is related to the number of subjects in the study. If enough subjects are employed, even a very small correlation (such as .10) may be statistically significant. Instead of this transformed value, most researchers evaluate the correlation using the coefficient of determination (to be discussed below).

Spearman Correlation (r_s)

The Spearman correlation is calculated on ranked or ordinal data. Raw scores or counts must be transformed into ranks before this test can be employed. A Spearman test might be performed to compare the order of finish for the Kentucky Derby and Belmont horse races. A perfect positive correlation would indicate identical orders of finish in the two races. A perfect negative correlation would indicate that the order of finish reversed itself. A correlation close to zero would indicate that knowing the order of finish for one race would provide no clues about the order of finish for the other.

The formula for calculation of the Spearman coefficient is:

$$r_s = 1 - \frac{6 \Sigma D^2}{N(N^2 - 1)}$$

Where D = difference scores
N = number of subjects (pairs of scores)

A difference score is calculated for each subject on the two measures and then squared. Remember the value must fall between -1 and $+1$.

Pearson Product-Moment Correlation

The Pearson correlation is calculated on raw data measures. The test specifically looks for a linear relationship between variables. Any other shape of relationship (even a perfect curvilinear relationship) will result in a correlation coefficient near zero. It is often wise to draw a scatter plot of data on graph paper using the two scores for each subject as co-ordinates in order to have an idea of the shape of the relationship. This will help you determine whether the Pearson is the appropriate test.

If there is a perfect linear correlation, the data points will form a straight line. Generally when you encounter the unmodified term *correlation* in a statistical context, reference is being made to the Pearson Product Moment (r).

$r = +1$ $r = -1$

The formula for the Pearson is presented in two forms. The conceptual formula consists of a quantity known as the sum of cross products divided by the square root of the product of the sum of squares for each of the two measures (X and Y). The more imposing formula on the right is simply the computation version.

$$r = \frac{\Sigma xy}{\sqrt{\Sigma x^2 \Sigma y^2}} \qquad r = \frac{\Sigma XY - \frac{(\Sigma X)(\Sigma Y)}{N}}{\sqrt{\left(\Sigma X^2 - \frac{(\Sigma X)^2}{N}\right)\left(\Sigma Y^2 - \frac{(\Sigma Y)^2}{N}\right)}}$$

Notice that all values are based on raw scores (capital letters) rather than interim calculations such as the sum of squares. The reasons that this is a safer formula for actual calculations have been discussed.

Before we move away from correlational techniques, one last observation about correlation and causation: Statistics tell us what happened — they *don't* tell us why. A correlation tells us that two variables covary. It does not tell us anything about causation, even in cases where there may actually be a causative relationship. There are more sophisticated techniques such as path analysis and confirmatory factor analysis that do begin to speak to the issue of causation. But, again, the basic forms of correlation coefficient do not.

□ LINEAR REGRESSION □

Linear regression provides another way of looking at the relationship between two measured variables. Whereas the correlation coefficient describes the relationship between the variables, in linear regression the goal is to develop the equation for the line that does the best job of describing the data.

If we draw a scatter plot of the data (using the two measures x and y for each subject as the coordinates for the point representing the subject), unless we have a perfect linear relationship the points will not fall precisely along a line. The challenge, then, is to find the line that is closest to the largest number of data points. If we consider distance of a point above our line as a positive deviation and distance below the line as negative deviation, we cannot calculate accuracy by simply adding distances from the line. Our values would cancel each other out. So (as we have done before with deviation scores), we square the values of the deviations and sum them. The best (most accurate) line will have the smallest sum for the squared deviations. Hence the name of the method — least squares.

Once we have the best line, we can use the equation to predict scores on one measure on the basis of scores on the other. Our measure of accuracy is the same measure commonly used for determining the practical value of correlations — the coefficient of determination.

The formula for a line is $Y = A + BX$. A represents the intercept, the point on the Y (vertical) axis where the line bisects the axis. B represents the slope of the line or the number of units on the Y axis the measure changes for each unit change on the X axis.

In linear regression our basic formula is $\hat{y} = a + bX$. In this case, $\hat{y}$ is the value we will predict for measure Y based on our knowledge of the relationship between the measures and the subject's score on measure X.

First, however, we must use our data to calculate a and b. The formula for b on the left is the conceptual formula.

$$b = \frac{\Sigma xy}{\Sigma x^2} = \frac{\Sigma XY - \dfrac{(\Sigma X)(\Sigma Y)}{N}}{\Sigma X^2 - \dfrac{(\Sigma X)^2}{N}}$$

If these formulas look familiar, glance back to the formulas for the Pearson correlation coefficient. Since what we are doing in both cases is dealing with the relationship between variables, it should not be surprising that the techniques are similar.

Finally, we employ the following formula to calculate *a*:

$$a = Y - bX$$

Where Y = mean of Y measures
X = mean of X measures

But wait. If we already have *Y* measures on subjects, why are we bothering to predict them? The comparison between the predicted value for *Y* for a subject and the actual value obtained on the measure by the subject gives us some idea about how well our equation describes the real relationship. There is a better way. We can calculate a coefficient of determination.

□ COEFFICIENT OF DETERMINATION (r^2). □

The coefficient of determination may be thought of as a measure of the practical value or accuracy of both Pearson correlation coefficients and linear regression equations. The coefficient of determination ranges in value from 0 to 1 and refers to the proportion of variability in one measure that we account for with the other measure. Another way of looking at it is that the coefficient of determination is equivalent to the proportion of variation that is eliminated in a linear regression if the regression equation is used to calculate predicted values for *Y*. Either way, large values are desirable. A coefficient of determination of .85 (the coefficient is usually expressed as a proportion) tells the researcher that only 15% of the variability in the research measures is unexplained by the observed relationship.

The calculation of the coefficient of determination for the Pearson correlation coefficient is absurdly simple. Look at the symbols for the statistics: *r* for the Pearson, r^2 for the coefficient of determination. Right! The obtained value for the correlation is simply squared. This will always result in a positive value for the coefficient of determination. Thus a correlation of -.95 (an almost perfectly inverse relationship) would have a coefficient of determination of .9025. Slightly over 90% of the variability is accounted for.

It was mentioned in our discussion of the Pearson that the coefficient of determination is often a more practical measure than the level of statistical significance. This is because the significance of the correlation is related to the number of subjects in the study. If there are enough subjects, a correlation of .10 may be statistically significant. When we calculate the coefficient of determination for this measure we see we are only accounting for 1% of the variability! Thus we are not accounting for 99%. In such a case it would seem clear that the coefficient of determination provides a vastly more useful piece of information.

The calculation of the coefficient of determination for a linear regression equation is slightly more complex. The formula includes two terms (b and the sum of the cross products) already calculated as part of the calculation of the equation. The denominator (the sum of squares for Y) is calculated using the

$$r^2 = \frac{b\Sigma xy}{\Sigma y^2}$$

Where b = slope calculated for linear regression
Σxy = sum of cross products (already calculated)
Σy^2 = sum of squares for Measure Y.

standard computational formula. The additional information supplied by the coefficient of determination far outweighs the effort required to calculate the single additional term.

□ MULTIPLE REGRESSION □

Few characteristics or variables associated with human beings have simple linear relationships. Almost always we can increase the accuracy of our prediction equation (raise our r^2) through the addition of more variables in the prediction equation. In multiple regression that is precisely what is done. Additional measures (predictor variables) are added to the equation in the hopes of increasing the accuracy of our predictions for variable Y. When we add these predictors our equation expands. A three-predictor equation would look like:

$$\hat{Y} = a + b_1X_1 + b_2X_2 + b_3X_3$$

Computationally this is much more complex than the linear regression case. We must calculate values for a (still the intercept) and three separate b values (the slopes of the lines for the relationship between this predictor and Y). In this case the calculation would involve the solution of three equations in three unknowns called "normal" equations. Don't worry. No one actually calculates multiple regressions. As you will see in Chapter 14, there are a number of useful computer packages that will perform the calculations.

Just as we measured the accuracy of the linear regression model with the coefficient of determination, so too we employ this measure in multiple regression, except here we label it R^2 as it represents multiple predictors. If we were to obtain an R^2 of .92 for an equation with three predictors (as illustrated above) it would tell us that all three together account for

92% of the variability in *Y*. But suppose we wanted to know how much of that 92% was being accounted for by predictor *X*? Unless we modify the multiple regression procedure, we can't tell.

A special procedure known as a stepwise regression solves our problem. The equation is first calculated using the single best predictor (determined as the predictor having the largest correlation with *Y*). An R^2 is determined for this first step. In the second step of the procedure the next best predictor is added to the equation so that the prediction equation consists of two predictors. An R^2 is calculated for the combination of the two predictors. However, since we already know how much variability was accounted for by the first predictor, if we subtract the first R^2 from the R^2 in step 2, we are left with the unique contribution of the second predictor. This stepwise process is continued, adding a new variable each time, until either no further gains in the R^2 occur or there are no more variables.

Multiple regression is quite a complex procedure. This discussion barely skims the surface. For further detail refer to a statistics text.

□ TIME SERIES ANALYSIS □

Uninterrupted time series are employed as the basis for describing historical data and forecasting future trends in the phenomena of interest. In simple uninterrupted time series data there has been no experimental manipulation or intervention.

For the time series model, the actual data measures (e.g., the number of occupational therapy patients seen in Anytown Hospital in June of 1986) are determined to consist of four components:

$$\text{Actual value} = \text{Trend} \times \text{Seasonal} \times \text{Cyclical} \times \text{Irregular}$$

Trend is a long-term gradual change in a measure. For example, the height of the average twelve-year-old American girl has increased steadily since the year 1900. Long-term evidence of consistent change allows for predictions of the phenomenon for the future.

The trend value for the data is calculated through regression procedures. First a linear regression model is fitted to the data to determine if the trend shows a straight line (linear) functional relationship. A multiple regression procedure attempts to fit a more complex shape to the trend. Through the comparison of the R^2 and r^2 (coefficients of determination), the more appropriate model can be identified.

Seasonal variation is based on periodic change that repeats within the course of the year. Many phenomena exhibit seasonal variation — for example, the average daily temperature, the number of spinal cord injuries sustained in diving accidents, or the number of children poisoned by eating mistletoe.

Seasonal variation is calculated in terms of seasonal indices. (Indices can be based on quarterly data or monthly data.) Seasonal indices vary around a base value of 100. A seasonal index of 100 indicates that this season experienced 100% of the variability associated with the "average" season. Thus an index of 100 shows no seasonal variation. (Quarterly seasonal indices must sum to 400, monthly indices to 1200.) These indices can be applied to actual measured data to "deseasonalize" the figure — remove the effect of the measure solely attributable to the time at which it occurred.

Cyclical variation is regular variability that occurs in periods longer than one year. This value is not calculated directly; rather the actual figures are adjusted by removing the other components, leaving the cyclical variation.

Irregular variability is any variation remaining when time series models have accounted for all they can. Irregular variability is unpredictable and gives forecasters nightmares. Any phenomenon with a large irregular variability component is extremely difficult to anticipate correctly.

□ INTERRUPTED TIME SERIES ANALYSIS □

Interrupted time series designs involve the introduction of an experimental manipulation or intervention into a series of measures of the dependent variable. The goal of analysis then is to determine the effectiveness of the intervention amidst the variability of the time series. The following discussion is based on the discussion by McCairn and McCleary in Cook and Campbell (1979).

Traditionally, regression models have been employed to analyze interrupted time series designs. McCairn and McCleary argue strongly against this usage on the grounds that for usual regression procedures (least squares) the error terms for the data points are assumed to be unrelated. This is probably not the case for interrupted time series data.

Instead, McCairn and McCleary recommend ARIMA (autoregressive integrated moving average) techniques in conjunction with models developed by Box and Jenkins (1976). Interrupted time series data consist of two components, the effect (or "deterministic" component) and the error (noise or "stochastic" component). The stochastic component can be further subdivided into systematic and unsystematic components. ARIMA techniques first make a model of the systematic stochastic component, then Box-Jenkins models are employed to evaluate the intervention.

The ARIMA procedures remove trend and seasonal variation from the data. Once an ARIMA model is completed, three different models known as "transfer functions" are tested. The first transfer function measures for abrupt, constant change; the second for gradual, constant change; and the third for abrupt, temporary change. In a manner similar to regression techniques, the ability of each of these models to predict scores for subjects is tested. If one of the models increases predictive ability above that of the ARIMA model alone, the intervention is judged effective. (Again, the reader is referred to other sources for a complete discussion of the procedure.)

□ SUMMARY □

Techniques for the analysis of data for quasi- and non-experimental research include the chi square tests, correlational techniques, linear regression, the coefficient of determination, multiple regression, time series analysis, and interrupted time series analysis.

Chi square tests are employed on nominal data to determine whether observed frequencies are similar to expected frequencies. The three types of chi square test are the simple chi square test, the contingency chi square test, and the "goodness of fit" test.

Correlational techniques allow the investigator to determine the extent of covariation between two variables. The Spearman correlation is applied to ordinal data and the Pearson Product-Moment correlation to ratio or interval data. Neither test allows for a statement of causation.

The regression techniques determine how accurately a variable may be described or predicted by knowledge of the values of one (linear regression) or more additional variables (multiple regression). The coefficient of determination allows for a statement of the actual amount of variability in the variables that is accounted for by their relationship.

Time series analysis examines the various components of observational data measures taken over a period of time. Trend represents gradual long-term change, seasonal variability represents changes in the measure explainable by the time of year of the measure, cyclical variability represents patterned variability in which the period of repetition exceeds one year, and irregular variability is any remaining fluctuation not accounted for by the first three components. Time series data are employed in forecasting.

Interrupted time series analysis seeks to evaluate the effectiveness of an experimental manipulation introduced in time series measures. The autoregressive integrated moving average (ARIMA) and Box-Jenkins modeling techniques allow for evaluation of the effect after the usual time series components are removed from the data.

□ KEY TERMS □

chi square test
simple chi square
contingency chi square
"goodness of fit" chi square
correlation
Spearman correlation
Pearson product-moment
   correlation
linear regression
coefficient of determination

multiple regression
stepwise regression
time series analysis
trend
seasonal variability
cyclical variability
irregular variability
interrupted time series
ARIMA (autoregressive integrated
   moving average)

□□ 14 □□

The Computer as a Research Tool

□ *Historical Overview*
□ *Computer Hardware*
□ *Computer Software*
□ *Computer Packages*
□ *Analyzing Your Data*
□ *Word Processing*

Computers are tremendously beneficial to researchers. Data analysis that at one time would have been extremely tedious and time-consuming can now be accomplished in a very short time. This chapter presents an overview of the development of computers and their applications in the research endeavor. No attempt will be made to present specific "how-to's" because at the speed computer software and hardware are changing, any such information would swiftly be rendered obsolete. However, a familiarity with the basic concepts and terms will ease the transition to the specific documentation that describes the actual procedures required in using specific computers or programs.

□ HISTORICAL OVERVIEW □

The first successful electronic computer—the Mark I—was completed by Howard Aiken of Harvard University in 1944. Thus began the revolution in the handling of data and information. Even the earliest computers represented a major increase in speed and accuracy over the calculations of human beings. The first-generation computers (1946) were, however, quite large. They depended on vacuum tubes and often occupied entire floors of buildings. Information was supplied to these early computers through either punched cards or tape at the site of the computer.

By 1959, the so-called second-generation computers appeared. These computers used transistors rather than vacuum tubes and were thus much more compact and could handle more information in a much smaller space. These smaller, faster units were also sometimes broken down into component parts rather than being one indivisible unit.

The third-generation computers of 1965 represented still another move in the direction of miniaturization. The use of integrated circuits allowed for yet smaller, extremely fast units. Technological advances allowed input of data from remote terminals and parallel processing of programs. (That is, the computer could do several calculations simultaneously rather than sequentially.) The so-called minicomputers were introduced, as were a number of new programming languages.

The development of the microprocessor in 1970 marked the beginning of the fourth generation of computers. The space required for a computer was now so small that home computers became a possibility, and as costs associated with the technology fell, these home computers became a major industry. A microcomputer central processing unit that cost $300 in 1971 had dropped in cost to $3 by 1982 (Isshiki, 1982). By this time American culture had accepted computerization so completely that computers were being used in all types of business and in many educational settings—even for children as young as pre-school age.

□ COMPUTER HARDWARE □

The term *hardware* refers to the physical components of the computer—the machine itself. Although there are a number of categories of computers (variously assigned by size or cost), from the largest mainframes to the smallest microcomputers, all consist of five basic components: (1) an input device, (2) a control unit, (3) an arithmetic-logic unit, (4) a storage unit, and (5) an output device.

There are many forms of input device. Basically this system acts as the ears of the computer. All data and programming commands enter the system through the input device. Larger and older computers often receive their data through cards or tapes.

Computer cards are heavy paper cards that contain 80 columns in which data may be placed. The data are literally punched into the cards as a pattern of holes by a keypunch machine, which has a typewriter-like keyboard and produces a "deck" (stack) of cards. The prepared card decks are fed into equipment known as card readers, which convey the information from the cards into the computer itself.

Card input is inefficient: Cards become expensive over the long run in terms of purchase price and storage space. An error made in punching a card can only be corrected by punching a whole new card. Furthermore, prepared decks have a disagreeable habit of falling all over the floor. For a long program this is a bit like having *War and Peace* typed line by line on 3-by-5 cards and having someone drop and scramble the cards. Because of these drawbacks and others, card input devices have been replaced by cathode ray tube (CRT) terminals. The cathode ray tube is much like (and often is) a television set attached to a typewriter-style keyboard. Information typed onto the screen is relayed to the computer. If any error is made in a data entry line it can be corrected on the spot.

Initially there was some adverse reaction to the introduction of CRT terminals into general use. There were questions (currently unresolved) about possible health hazards—some potentially severe. Eyestrain and headaches were attributed to the use of terminals, as were alleged increases in the rate of birth defects and miscarriages among pregnant women whose work required the use of terminals.

The input device (card reader or terminal) sends the input information into the central processing unit (CPU), which consists of the control unit and the arithmetic-logic unit. The control unit (as the name implies) does not actually process information. Rather, it controls the other units in the computer in order to execute the program. The arithmetic-logic unit actually handles all processing of data, including all calculations and decisions. It is the size of the CPU that has changed dramatically as computers have evolved.

Data and programs may be stored in the computer in what is known as computer memory. The information is recorded magnetically on tapes or disks. There are two main types of disk, hard and floppy, which are generally used in different systems. Both tapes and disks can be stored outside the computer and reintroduced when required.

The output unit provides feedback on what the computer has processed. When the input device is a terminal, often that same terminal serves as the output device. The results of data analysis are flashed on the screen. This is often not sufficient, however, for the researcher who would like to have a "hard" (printed) copy of the results. For this documentation an earlier form of output device is still employed. High-speed printers reproduce the information provided on the CRT screen; in a system that employs card readers, the printer may stand alone as the sole output device.

□ COMPUTER SOFTWARE □

The term *hardware* denotes the mechanical components of the computer described above. The machine must be instructed as to what to do, however. Instructions are given through *software*, or programs. Software can be divided into two categories: systems software and applications software.

Systems software is the basic level at which the computer is given commands. Computers don't speak English, they speak machine language. Essentially they only respond to commands that are presented in a numerical code. The earliest computer machine languages were in binary code. More recent languages have used octal or hexidecimal codes. These languages are machine-specific in that they provide specific, minutely detailed commands to a specific CPU hardware system. IBM machine language is thus different from that of a Univac or DEC computer. Almost no one actually employs machine language in using a computer. Programming languages have been developed that are easier for humans to use; the computer internally translates these into machine language for its own use.

Applications software communicates to the computer the desired commands for performing a particular piece of processing. Applications software is written in languages much more "user-friendly" (adapted to the cognitive idiosyncrasies of human beings) than machine language. Letters and words are used in several layers of languages. Each step away from the basic simplicity of machine language requires the computer to translate commands. There are several successive layers of languages. Thus, if a high-level language is employed, the computer may be required to make several successive translations.

The lowest level of applications software is assembly language, or assembler. Assembly languages can be thought of as the English equivalent of machine language. Instructions are still extremely detailed. For example you can't, in assembly language, just tell the computer to add 2 + 2. You must tell it where to go to get the first number, where to hold it while it retrieves the second, what to do with the two numbers, and what to do with the result.

Symbolic languages (also known as high-level languages) do not require such detail. When the computer translates from a symbolic language to assembly to machine languages, these machine-oriented instructions are inserted automatically as part of the translation process. Symbolic languages have been developed for a number of specific applications. FORTRAN, one of the earliest high-level languages, is essentially a mathematical-scientific language primarily useful in computations—data analysis, for example. A number of more recent languages, such as BASIC, PASCAL, APL, or PL/1, could also be employed (depending on the computer being used). Although FORTRAN has undergone a number of revisions and simplifications, the newer languages tend to be easier to learn and use.

Irrespective of the language used, programming instructions for the analysis of data (in other words, the mathematics) must be conveyed to the computer along with the data itself. Fortunately, a number of computer packages have been written that enable a researcher with virtually no knowledge of programming to conduct computerized data analysis.

□ COMPUTER PACKAGES □

Computer packages represent the farthest distance away from machine language. Packages are written in such a way that rather than instructions having to be given for each step in the equations for an analysis, a single statement such as "PROC MREG"(from SAS, 1982) will tell the computer to perform a multiple regression analysis on a data set. Thus, all the researcher really needs to know is the statistical procedure that should be used and how to input the data. Actually, the process is a bit more complicated than that. The researcher must familiarize himself or herself with the capabilities of the package to be employed, and have a basic level of familiarity with the use of computers.

There are essentially three generally useful packages available to researchers without computer programming skills: (1) SAS (1982), (2) SPSS (1975, 1981) and SPSSX (1983), and (3) BMDP (1981). (Let us hasten to add that these packages are so good that many researchers *with* programming skills also use them.) In addition, there are a number of more esoteric packages. For example, Multivariance (1978) calculates only analysis of variance procedures. The general programs contain descriptive and inferential statistical procedures commonly employed in data analysis. SAS is most often encountered in business settings because it is especially useful for handling files and writing reports. SPSS and BMDP are more commonly encountered in educational and hospital settings.

□ ANALYZING YOUR DATA □

If you had a set of data to analyze, how would you go about it? If you are affiliated with an institution of higher learning or a hospital you probably have access to a computer center. Locating the center is your first step. In order to use time on a computer you must pay for it somehow. This can be done with actual money in the case of individuals not affiliated with the computer center's institution, or with credits if you are affiliated. In either case you need an account in your name or access to an account with funds.

Once you have an account you will be provided with information that will allow you to log onto the system. Usually this involves telling the system your name, your account number, and your password. Your password is the key to your account. Without the proper password, no one but you can access the account. If you are working from a terminal the log-on will allow you to set up the files you will need for analysis. If you use cards, a log-on equivalent will be the first card on your deck.

Because computers and computer centers vary so widely, the best advice at this point would be to cultivate the staff of the center—known as consultants. They will help you to find the documentation explaining how to employ the packages as well as how to do such basics as turn on the terminal and direct your output to a printer. Many people are intimidated by computers and computer-type people. Remember, once upon a time they didn't know anything either. It's their job to help you.

One final word on data analysis. If you do not have experience with computers, expect the process at first to be tedious, intimidating, and sometimes frustrating. Computers are dumb. They must be told *exactly* what to do, and an unexpected space or comma may confuse the computer terribly. It takes a while to adjust to the level of precision necessary. But hang on. Even with hitches the computer will achieve in minutes what would take you and your calculator a week to accomplish!

□ WORD PROCESSING □

Another advance the computer age has provided is the capability of word processing. Word processing is typing on the computer. Almost all microcomputers have word-processing software, as do almost all mainframe systems. Word processing on a computer terminal allows you to correct your errors before printing up your report and to store the report for later reentry to edit. This means that changes can be made without the whole document having to be retyped. Computer word-processing is a blessing for those who type well and a miracle for those who don't. Consult your computer center for further information.

□ SUMMARY □

The computer has become an almost indispensible research aid. Computer hardware has advanced to the point where home computers are commonplace. The computer itself consists of the *input device*, which reads data into the *central processing unit*, which in turn consists of the *control unit* and the *arithmetic-logic unit* where data processing actually takes place. Calculations and information are placed in the *memory unit*, where they may be accessed to provide feedback to the researcher through an *output unit*. Data analysis that would require large amounts of time without a computer can be completed in several minutes with the computer. Word processing computer capabilities have vastly simplified the preparation of reports.

Software is the term for the directions given to the computer. Systems software represents the very basic command level and is in numerical code. Applications software consists of languages that tell the computer what computations are desired. Symbolic languages are high-level program languages such as FORTRAN that facilitate human-computer interactions. These languages have been organized into "packages," such as SAS, SPSSX, or BMDP, that allow the non-programming investigator to direct the computer data analyses.

□ KEY TERMS □

input device
control unit
arithmetic-logic unit
storage unit
output device
keypunch
cathode ray tube (CRT)

central processing unit (CPU)
software
systems software
applications software
assembly language
symbolic language

□□ 15 □□
Communicating Research

- ■ *Abstract*
- □ *Introduction*
- □ *Methods*
- □ *Results*
- □ *Style*
- □ *Communicating With Tables and Figures*
- □ *References*
- □ *Funding Sources and Publication Outlets*
- □ *Publishing Research Reports*

The world's most startlingly innovative research or most brilliant ideas are worthless if they are not communicated well. The purpose of the research report is to allow others in the discipline, especially those interested in research, access to the most current information in the field.

The general format of research reports is fairly standard across the health science professions. The order is very much that presented in this text. An Abstract is followed by an Introduction, a Methods section, a Results section, a Discussion of the results, and a listing of References.

□ ABSTRACT □

The abstract of a journal article is a short (generally approximately 100 words) summary of the entire study. When you're leafing through a journal issue, a glance at the abstract allows you to decide whether you want to read the entire article. The abstract contains one or two sentences representing the other sections of the article. From the introduction comes a brief statement of why the study was conducted. A one- or two-sentence summary of the methods section states how the procedures were implemented and upon whom. The results summary briefly indicates what was found. The summary of the discussion interprets the results. The reference section is not represented in the abstract.

Writing a good abstract is an art. You must be succinct without being so cryptic that the reader cannot understand what happened. After reading a well-written abstract you should have a good idea of the framework of the study. Because the abstract often appears not only in the journal with the article but also in the abstract collections discussed in Chapter 1, it is important to incorporate any key words or phrases associated with your particular type of research. As a consumer of the literature you will find these "buzz words" (key words) useful when using an abstract to decide whether to seek out a particular article.

□ INTRODUCTION □

The introduction section sets out the purpose of the study and a statement of the researcher's hypotheses and outcome predictions for the study. It may include a literature review if there is no separate literature section. The introduction should make a case for the study. In other words, evidence should be presented that supports the proposed procedures as well as the proposed hypotheses and predictions.

At times there will not exist a body of research literature in your topic area. In that case the literature review may be quite brief and may lean heavily on theoretical articles or model statements. For this type of study the hypotheses follow from logical extension of the theory. This is perfectly acceptable. In fact, to a lesser degree this also occurs in research where there is a body of literature. The important consideration is that all hypotheses are based on something, and it is important to be aware of any assumptions that are being used in the construction of hypotheses and predictions. This kind of analytical self-consciousness is not easy and is the hallmark of the good researcher. Regardless of the manner in which the hypotheses are derived, after reading the introduction the reader should have a clear understanding of why this research is being conducted, what outcomes are anticipated, and what the reasons for these expectations are.

□ METHODS □

The methods section contains the actual research design. Everything you need to know about subjects, equipment, and procedures should be contained in this section. For uncomplicated studies the information will be sufficient to allow you to repeat or replicate the study in your own setting. (For more complex studies you must often contact the author(s) for further details, plans for special equipment, or copies of questionnaires.) When writing a methods section, then, a good question to keep in mind is: "If I wanted to conduct this study, what facts would I need?"

Research subjects should be described in enough detail that a matching sample may be selected. This is not to say that the subjects' anonymity is violated or that tremendous amounts of space are taken up with irrelevant details, but any characteristics that are (or might be) important to the results of the study should be catalogued. Often these will include such characteristics as gender, age, diagnosis, or extent of chronicity. In addition, sampling procedures should be explained. In other words, who were the subjects and how were they obtained?

The methods section also contains a detailed description of the equipment and procedures employed. If a placebo or double blind procedure (Chapter 9) was used, how was it implemented? What kinds of equipment were used? Here you should specify not only the type of equipment, but the actual equipment (brand name and model number) employed.

Besides allowing for accurate replication, a detailed methods section can also prove helpful in evaluating the design and interpreting the results of research. The methods section (as well as the introduction) should be completed before the study is conducted. In fact, a methods section detailing procedures to be conducted is an integral part of a research proposal to be submitted to ethics committees or funding sources. Having to record the planned study forces attention to details that might otherwise be overlooked. Since control is an important issue in research, the forethought necessary to complete the methods section allows you to anticipate and prepare for various situations that might arise.

One of the realities of research (and life) is that things don't always turn out the way we expect or desire. Sometimes careful examination of the methods section will allow either the researcher or another reader to identify possible sources of disconfirmation of hypotheses. This use of a somewhat more objective colleague is strongly recommended before a study is conducted as well as after the fact. Researchers often become so close to and so involved with their study that they may begin to overlook assumptions they might be making, omissions or biases in research procedure, or lack of clarity in the research report.

□ RESULTS □

The results section reports on the statistical procedures employed to analyze the data and the outcomes in terms of statistical significance. For each statistical test there is a convention as to what information is reported.

Generally this involves stating the level of significance of the obtained statistic, the value of the statistic itself, and whatever additional information is necessary for the reader to evaluate the significance of the statistic (i.e., the number of subjects or the degrees of freedom). Stated another way, the reader should be able (on the basis of the information provided) to employ standardized tables to determine the level of significance of the obtained statistic.

Since the statement of statistical results can become confusing very quickly, tables and graphs are often employed to summarize and clarify the information. A more detailed discussion of these methods will appear later in this chapter.

In many ways, writing the results section is the most challenging part of the research report. Results must be presented in sufficient detail to communicate the outcomes of the study while at the same time being sufficiently simple so that the less statistically sophisticated reader will not be either confused or intimidated. Suprisingly enough, writing a comprehensible results section is often particularly a problem for the statistics wizards of the research world.

□ DISCUSSION □

The discussion section seeks to explain the significance of the results, to analyze reasons for the results, to qualify the results, and to speculate about the next step in this line of research. The purpose is really to tie up any and all loose ends.

But wait. Wasn't the purpose of the results section to explain the significance of the results? Yes and no. The results section deals with significance in the highly specific sense of statistical significance discussed in Chapter 11. As you will recall, this deals with the probability of our obtaining this result if, in fact, there was no effect. (How likely is it we would obtain this finding by chance?) In the discussion section we are talking about interpreting this statistical information in real world terms. The discussion section translates results from statistics to concepts, explanations, and possibly applications. Now that we have this information, what does it mean and what can we do with it? Sometimes we might cite literature not previously cited in the introduction in order to support our explanations.

Even when the results of the study achieve an acceptable level of significance we cannot be totally sure of our effect. Recall that with an alpha level of .05 there is still a 5% possibility that the effect does not in fact exist (Chapter 11). Therefore we must state our results in a somewhat tentative manner. Phrases such as "...it would appear that..." or "...would seem to indicate..." are frequently encountered in discussion sections. We can state with certainty what happened, but we can never be sure why we obtained our results. Appropriate research design helps by eliminating plausible rival explanations, but we can never escape the possibility of a Type I error. So be forceful in the statement of your statistical outcomes, but cautious in your interpretations.

Another important role of the discussion section is to recognize limitations of the study. Unfortunately, flaws in reasoning or design are often more obvious after the fact. Discussing what could be done differently in a future study helps to clarify the results or eliminate plausible alternative explanations for them.

Finally, the discussion section should consider the next step in the line of research. Whether or not the hypotheses were confirmed, each study adds a little more information to the common body of knowledge. Given the additional knowledge provided by this study, what next?

□ REFERENCES □

The final section of the paper lists the literature cited in the other sections. The reference section varies more widely in format than any other section of the report.

Given that the health science professions encompass a number of different disciplines, it is not surprising that there is not close agreement on the style to be employed in citing references. Indeed, it is surprising that the general format for research reports varies so little across not only the health sciences but also the social and behavioral sciences. However, there are almost as many styles for references as there are professional journals.

All the health sciences do share one requirement. For a reference to be listed, it must be cited in the body of the text. Whenever any idea is taken from another individual it must be so noted, and appropriate credit must be given. On the other hand, books or articles that stimulated your thoughts but from which you do not borrow citable ideas are not to appear in the reference section. The rules for references are very detailed and inflexible. It is necessary to be most painstaking in their preparation.

The discipline of physical therapy has adopted the most consistent style for references. The American Physical Therapy Association publishes a style manual that covers all possible situations. Not all journals in physical therapy employ this exact style, however, so if you are considering writing for publication it is safest to check first with the journal before proceeding.

The discipline of nursing has not accepted a single dominant style for references. Various styles are accepted, and different journals require different formats. In cases where a style is not imposed by a journal, three different styles appear to be about equally accepted. These styles are the format used in psychology and published in a style manual by the American Psychological Association (1983), and the styles in manuals by Turabian (1973) and Linton (1972).

Two different styles for references are employed in publications in the discipline of occupational therapy. The *Occupational Therapy Journal of Research* employs the format of the American Psychological Association (1983). The *American Journal of Occupational Therapy* publishes an *Author's Style Guide* (1979) governing references appearing in this journal.

□ STYLE □

The research report is a formal document. As such, it utilizes not only conventions for format but also a formal, conventional writing style.

It should be clearly pointed out at this juncture that the style of this text is much too informal and unconventional for a research report. This decision was made deliberately for a very clear reason. The topic of research itself often serves to intimidate students. It was felt that a first-person, extremely informal style and tone would help to demystify the concepts and render the entire topic more palatable. When research reports are being submitted to professional journals, however, there exist standards that must be met if the paper is to be accepted for publication. In addition to the discussion below, go to the major journals in your discipline (*Physical Therapy*, or *American Journal of Occupational Therapy*). Read through several articles or several issues. When writing research reports, emulate the style employed in your major journal. Always employ the third person for pronouns. Never use contractions.

The intent of the research report is to communicate research results. It is not to demonstrate the breadth of your vocabulary (or your facility with the thesaurus), your ability to write complex sentences, your statistical wizardry, your IQ, your charm, or your wit. Again, your goal is to communicate. The reader should not have to struggle to understand what you're trying to say. Or struggle through excess verbiage to find your point. (If you attempt to publish, one of your first rude shocks will probably involve the extreme brevity demanded by editors!)

It is vital, then, that your report be clear, simple, direct, and brief. Clarity can often be enhanced through the use of simple language and sentence structure. Simple declarative sentences should be the rule. Basic terminology should be employed. Don't worry if one term appears so many times you feel it is redundant, particularly in the methods and results sections. It happens. Particularly in these sections, clarity is vastly more important than "style."

Be as brief as possible without sacrificing comprehensiveness and clarity. As you recall from Chapter 2, one of the hallmarks of a good theory is parsimony. The same holds true for research reports, particularly if you aspire to publication.

It should be clear that principles of good English should be followed. Verb tenses should be consistent; generally the past tense is used. Rules of grammar should be observed. Punctuation should be carefully checked. Used correctly, punctuation adds clarity. Misused it obscures meaning. Most often abused is the comma. A common error is to use the comma far too liberally. If your sentences are brief and direct enough you should not need a lot of commas. When in doubt, look it up or don't use it.

After you have written up a research report, it is often useful to ask a colleague to critique the report for content and style. First, however, try to read it yourself with a detached attitude. (Often setting it aside for several days enhances objectivity.) Ask yourself whether, solely on the basis of what is written and without any reliance on your special knowledge, you can understand what the report is about. What about the style? If it seems boring and redundant to you, you are probably close to the necessary style required by editors.

□ COMMUNICATING WITH TABLES AND FIGURES □

As stated above, the clear communication of statistical results is particularly challenging. Results are usually presented both in the text itself and in some sort of tabular or graphic form.

Tables are used primarily to summarize data. Chapter 10 dealt with frequency distributions, which present raw data in summary form. Frequency distributions are often presented in conjunction with the mean and standard deviation to provide the reader with a description of the measures.

Another specialized form of table, known as a source table, is used in conjunction with the statistical technique known as the analysis of variance (ANOVA). Tables of this kind summarize the calculations of the statistic for each source of variability in the research design. Chapter 12 contains a more comprehensive discussion of ANOVA.

In using tables to summarize statistical data there are a number of issues to bear in mind. It is very important to include the value of the obtained statistic and the significance level of the statistic. There is a tendency to include too much information in tables. In this case less is definitely more. The intent of tables is to simplify the reader's task, therefore it is pointless to design a table that overwhelms with information.

Keep tables simple and clear. Spread out the information and make use of open space to highlight your results. If the table seems at all crowded, consider dividing the information into several smaller tables. Also consider the visual balance and aesthetics of the table. It should be uncluttered and readily interpretable.

Tables can only be easily interpreted if they are clearly labeled. Every table should have a title that clearly identifies the content of the table. Each column in the table should have a column heading. Although novice researchers tend to crowd the contents of tables, they also tend to underlabel. On completing a table you should ask yourself: "Would this make sense if I were not familiar with this study?" In other words, do you have to have special knowledge beyond what is available in the table in order to understand the information? Another extremely useful technique is to show it to a colleague who isn't familiar with the study and solicit feedback.

Another approach to summarizing data involves the use of graphs, also known as figures. Graphics provide a dramatic summary of results and should be considered even when the data are simple enough to preclude the use of tables—the explosion in the availability of graphic software for computers has made it easy to present quantitative information in graphic form.

Certain kinds of graphs are particularly suited for specific types of studies. For nominal data (see Chapter 2) bar charts or pie charts may be employed. Pie charts (Fig. 15-1) are generally used when the data consist of proportions or percentages of a population or sample figure. The figures in

Anytown Hospital: Age at Admission, November 1981

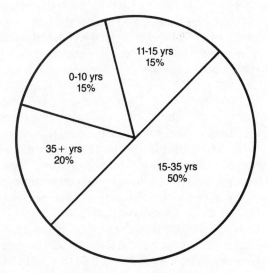

FIGURE 15-1   Example of a pie chart.

the segments of the chart should sum to 1.00 or 100%. If necessary, include a "Miscellaneous" category to complete the whole.

Labeling is also an important consideration for graphics. The reader should understand clearly not only what the entire chart represents but also what each segment stands for.

Bar charts belong to a family of graphic representations known as histograms. A histogram consists of two axes set at 90° angles to each other. The vertical axis is known as the ordinate (*y* axis) and the horizontal axis is known as the abscissa (*x* axis).

Each axis is divided into unit measures. The ordinate represents values or frequencies of the measures in the study. Along the abscissa are represented the various categories (for nominal data) or scores obtainable by subjects. By convention, the point at which the axes meet is known as the origin and represents a value of zero on both axes. Points to the right of or above the origin represent positive values; points to the left of or below the origin indicate negative values.

If your range of data values begins well above zero, convention requires you to slash the lines as shown in Figure 15-2*A* to indicate the break in numerical continuity from the origin. Aesthetically, it is generally best to draw a histogram so that it is three quarters as high (tall) as it is long (wide).

When bar charts are used to illustrate nominal data, the bars on the chart represent data categories. Figure 15-2*B* summarizes data on the types of cases dealt with by an occupational therapy department during the course of a year. The bars do not touch each other because the categories are discrete (Chapter 2). Figure 15-2*A* represents continuous data (in this case, patient age). For continuous measures, the class boundary is used to divide the data into classes. The area of the bar is equal to the frequency of the category. If all categories (classes) are of equal width, then height on the ordinate indicates frequency. If one category is twice as wide as others, however, its height must be proportionally smaller, as can be seen in Figure 15-3

Another frequently useful form of graphic representation is known as the frequency polygon. As with the bar chart, the frequency polygon allows you to compare frequencies of category membership. But the frequency polygon is useful in illustrating more complex data. For example, if we were interested in subdividing the information in Figure 15-2*B* into case type as a function of gender, a bar chart could become quite busy and difficult to read. Use of two separate bar charts (or pie charts) defeats the purpose of making any direct comparisons.

A frequency polygon represents data categories with a point rather than a bar. The value of the point is the class mark. The height on the ordinate is the frequency of that class. Points for category of interest (i.e. female patients) are connected and carefully labeled. The lines representing

Anytown Hospital, November, 1986.
Age of Osteoporosis Patients

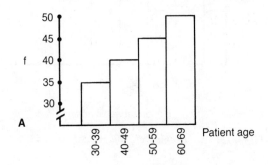

A

Patient age

Anytown Hospital, 1981.
Patients seen in Department of Occupational Therapy.

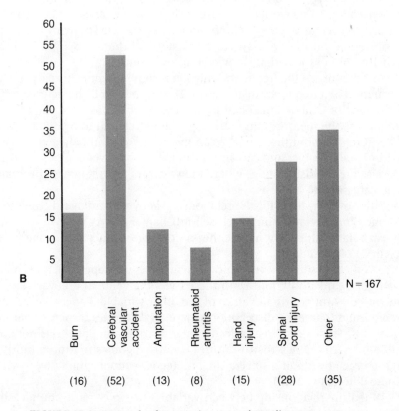

B

N = 167

FIGURE 15-2   *Example of* (A) *continuous and* (B) *discrete measures.*

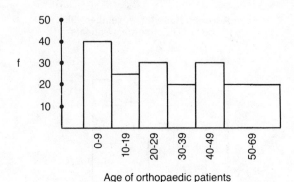

FIGURE 15-3   Example of proportional class widths.

our male patient categories and our female patient categories can be directly compared.

A frequency polygon is also very useful in illustrating a change in time where elapsed time would be measured along the abscissa, while a clinical measure (such as degrees of limb mobility or muscle strength) would be represented on the ordinate, and the slope of the line would indicate whether or not the patient showed improvement.

Another use of the frequency polygon is to represent pictorially the information in a frequency distribution. There are several characteristic distributions of data as illustrated by frequency polygons. (For the sake of simplicity, the measures on both axes will be referred to below as variables. Keep in mind that *variable* can mean the relation between two experimental variables and can also mean the pictorial version of a measure on afrequency distribution, where the variables are frequency [ordinate] and category or class [abscissa]).

The simplest shape for the relationship between variables is the monotonic, linear relationship discussed in Chapter 13. As you will recall, a linear relationship may have either a positive or a negative slope, as in Figure 15-4 *A* and *B*.

Another possible linear relationship involves no slope at all and can be seen in Figure 15-4 *C* and *D*. In these cases the value of one variable remains constant across all values of the other variable. Panel *C* could also represent a frequency distribution where all categories display equal frequencies. This is known as a rectangular distribution. Panel *D* is not possible for a frequency distribution. (The analogous situation would be represented by a point, since a single category cannot simultaneously assume different values.)

When the relationship between variables becomes more complex the resulting pictorial representation can no longer be represented by a simple

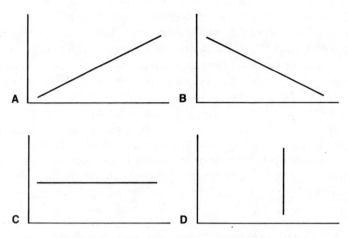

FIGURE 15-4   *Examples of linear relationships.*

equation. Two characteristic distributions, as seen in Figure 15-5, are the U-shaped and the "normal" distribution.

The U-shaped (or inverted U-shaped) distribution results when the relationship between variables is best described by a quadratic equation. This shape is characteristic of an interaction effect in an analysis of variance (where the values of variable *X* are differentially responsive to values of variable *Y* [Chapter 12]).

The normal distribution is characteristic of the frequency distributions of many naturally occurring phenomena such as human height, weight, and IQ. The mathematical equation describing the normal curve is complex because at points equidistant from the midpoint the shape of the curve changes from convex to concave. These "deflection points" occur exactly one standard deviation unit above and below the mean. In data that have a normal distribution, the mean, median, and mode all have the same value. The normal distribution also possesses some very useful mathematical qualities, as you learned (or will learn) in your statistics training.

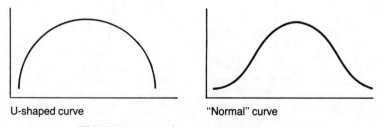

U-shaped curve   "Normal" curve

FIGURE 15-5   *U-shaped and normal curves.*

Distributions can also be categorized by the comparative shapes of the distribution on either side of the midpoint. Distributions are considered symmetric if the sides of the distribution, when hypothetically peeled off the page and folded at midpoint, match each other in shape. Rectangular, U-shaped, and normal distributions are symmetric; linear relationships are not.

It is possible to have an asymmetric curvilinear relationship, as can be seen in Figure 15-6. The off-balance nature of the curve is referred to as *skew*. Panel A illustrates positive skew, while Panel B represents negative skew. (Memory hint: the skew is labeled by the direction in which the low-frequency end or "tail" points.) These terms are useful in the description of your figures as part of the text of your results section.

□ FUNDING SOURCES AND PUBLICATION OUTLETS □

Research can be an expensive proposition. Your time, materials or equipment used, possible financial incentives to subjects, and computer time for statistical analyses all cost money. Fortunately, you are not always forced

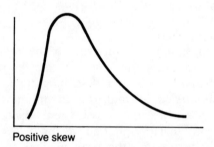

Positive skew

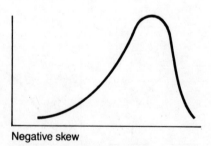

Negative skew

FIGURE 15-6   *Skew.*

to bear the costs alone. Government agencies such as the National Institutes for Health (NIH), agencies such as the National Science Foundation (NSF), and professional organizations can either provide funds or direct you to the sources of available funding.

When an agency has money available and an interest in a particular topic, they issue what is known as a call for proposals. In this document they specify their area of interest, stating the types of problems or content areas considered appropriate. Generally they will also specify the amount available per grant and administrative information such as how many copies of the proposal are to be submitted to whom. A final date for submission is included.

Requests for proposals are disseminated as widely as possible to the appropriate professional groups. Educational institutions, because of their research orientation, generally receive copies, as do directors of clinical training or research in clinical settings. Copies are also available on request from the agencies themselves.

Although requirements may vary somewhat, research proposals generally follow a standardized format. This format is an abbreviated form of the research report. In an introduction section you must convince the granting agency that you are familiar with the topic area and you must justify your proposed study through the use of a literature review. Just as in the introduction for the research report, you must state your hypotheses and predict your expected results. The goal of the research report is to communicate/sell ideas and knowledge. In the research proposal you are selling your plans to potential investors. You must convince them through a professional proposal that you represent a good risk for their funds. A well-written, comprehensive introduction can go a long way to establishing your perceived competence. The time you invest will not be wasted, particularly if you do receive funding. After you have conducted the research using their money, the granting agency will expect a research report to account for the funds. A well- written introduction often will require no modification for the final report.

The methods section of a proposal is very like a future-tense version of the methods section for the research report. Here you explain what you plan to do in enough detail to enable the granting agency reviewers to evaluate your proposed study. Because of the evaluation aspect you should probably spend more time and space explaining the reasons for your choices of subjects, procedure, and equipment than would be necessary in a final research report. Justify why choices you have made are the ones that best help you answer the research question. Give reasons why you have rejected other methods.

The major departure from the research report format in the research proposal is the budget proposal. You must request a specific amount of money and provide justifications as to why you require this particular amount.

Unfortunately, a certain amount of strategy is involved in writing a budget proposal quite apart from the actual need for funds. In the 1970s granting agencies reduced their financial support for research. As funds became short, some agencies attempted to continue funding a number of projects (rather than concentrating funds in a few places) by cutting proposed budgets by a flat percentage. For example, all funded studies would receive only 80% of the funds requested. Investigators promptly responded with inflated budgets. If you felt you really needed $50,000 and you knew the agency would cut your request by 20%, you requested $62,000. Such inflation often resulted in agencies making further cuts. Such game-playing was, and is, most common for requests for large amounts of money.

The budget should be broken down by category of expense. If salaries are requested over a period of time you should specify the amount of increase calculated for each successive year and separate out the figures for benefits or indirect personnel costs. Agencies will often provide you with an allowable figure for such costs (as a percentage of direct salary expense). If not, use the figure employed by your organization for such calculations. (The figure should be available from either the Personnel Office—Salary Administration division or the office dealing with contracts and grants for your institution.)

Figures for supplies should be based on current consumption. Actual costs of equipment as taken from price catalogues or brochures should be used. Be sure to think carefully of all possible expenses. It is probable your institution will demand a share of the grant for administrative costs. This "overhead" figure will be provided to you by the institution and usually consists of some percentage of the total budget figure excluding equipment costs.

Another important section of a grant proposal in the health sciences is the guarantee of ethical behavior and treatment of subjects. Considering the issues raised in Chapter 9, how can you ensure the protection of your subjects? Standards for research ethics have become more stringent over the years. Subjects must be guaranteed protection or the research should not be conducted. Most educational institutions have formed ethics committees that must approve the research proposal (regardless of any request for outside funding) before any application may be submitted or research conducted.

The preceding represents a brief summary of procedures for applying for grant funds. For more complete information, contact the granting agencies, the office at your institution responsible for administering grants, and locate one of the many how-to books on grantsmanship available.

□ PUBLISHING RESEARCH REPORTS □

Once you have completed your research you are ready to share your results with the world. It is now time to consider how you go about achieving publication in a professional journal.

The first step is to decide on the journal to which you will submit your manuscript. Journals take different positions on the types of studies and articles they will consider publishing. Some are oriented toward basic research, some focus more on clinical applications, some welcome purely theoretical work, others will not consider non-experimental work. So how do you know?

In each issue or volume of journals there appears a section entitled something along the lines of "Instructions to Authors." This contains information on the philosophical approach of the journal as well as directly practical information on such things as required margin sizes and reference format. Read carefully the information on the type of articles considered for publication. Unless you are sure your article fits the description, don't waste your time submitting your work to this particular journal. Continue looking. Different journals coexist because of their disparate foci. Choose the publication most likely to give your work serious consideration.

As you prepare your manuscript, be meticulous in your attention both to detail and to the authors' instructions. Be especially careful with the references. In order to discourage the tactic of sending copies of the same article to different journals for consideration, journals often adopt an idiosyncratic style for references. This means you would at least have to redo your references for multiple submission. (Actually, multiple submission is not considered professional behavior. It is much safer—as well as more ethical—to submit to journals sequentially if necessary.)

Once you have submitted the requested number of copies to the address indicated, you must sit back and wait—often for several months. While you are either going on with your life or chewing your nails, your paper is going through the review process. Acknowledged experts in the subject area of your paper will be given copies to read and critique. Sometimes the reviewers will be aware of the authorship of the paper. Since this can introduce a source of bias in which big names would automatically get published and beginners would have trouble regardless of the quality of the paper, a "blind" review process is often employed. In this process all identifying information is removed from the paper before it is seen by a reviewer.

The reviewer provides the journal's editors with a recommendation for the fate of the paper as well as a copy of the critique. "Good" reviewers often conduct such painstaking reviews that they will list typos, or suggest a change of wording in a section of the paper. Several reviewers will independently evaluate your study. The journal editor will consider all recommendations before making a decision. Occasionally, a paper will be sent to still further reviewers if the decision is still not clear.

Basically, your paper may be accepted, accepted with revisions, or rejected. Occasionally, an editor will reject a paper as it stands but encourage resubmission of a revised paper. If you are unequivocally accepted, celebrate and be justifiably proud of yourself. It doesn't happen very often.

If you are accepted with revisions or rejected you will usually be provided with copies of the reviewers' comments (no information will be given about the reviewers' identities). If you must make revisions, these comments often prove useful. Sometimes knowing the basis for rejection will provide you with ammunition to fight for reversal of the decision. Some reviewers with only rudimentary knowledge of an area such as statistics will nonetheless feel compelled to criticize your work. Sometimes they're wrong. If so, and you can prove it to the editor, and the rejection of your work was based on this reviewer's opinion, the decision may be changed. If the misunderstanding is based on your less-than-optimal communication of your ideas, you can restate your position. When you revise and resubmit your article the review process will be repeated. Whether or not the same reviewers are used depends on the journal.

If you are accepted (either initially or after revision) you are now officially "in press." Once the article has been set in type you will be sent a copy to proofread. This is not the time to make substantive changes: your changes should be confined to the correction of typos or small errors in printing. At this time you will usually be able to order copies of the reprinted article. These are not free (here's another cost to include in your grant proposal!). Some journals also charge you a portion of the costs associated with publishing the journal. Finally, after what seems like forever, the great day arrives and you have in your hands an issue of a journal containing your article. Congratulations! Add the entry to your curriculum vitae and head back to work.

□ SUMMARY □

The final step in the research process is sharing the results with the professional community through the use of formal reports published in journals devoted to the health-science disciplines. The general format required in such publications involves an abstract followed by an introduction, a methods section, a results section, a discussion section, and a listing of references.

The abstract is a very short precis of the entire article. Such abstracts may appear in collections of abstracts to be found in the reference section of the library. The introduction contains the statement of purpose of the study as well as the hypotheses to be studied and predicted outcomes. Previous research may be cited in a literature review to justify and support the present study.

The methods section contains information on the actual study. Subjects, equipment or data collection instruments, and procedures employed in data collection are described. The results section reports on the outcomes of the analyses of data in the study. Statistical procedures and results are presented, often in tabular or graphic form.

The discussion section seeks to explain the significance of the findings of the study. Any limitations of the study and recommendations for future research are also included. The references section cites the sources of literature presented in the report. The format for references varies across disciplines and publication outlets.

Research may be an expensive proposition. Various funding agencies supply grants of funds to support research in various fields. The format for applications for grant funds resembles that of the research report but describes the research in the future tense, as a proposal.

□ KEY TERMS □

abstract	bar charts
methods	pie charts
results	histogram
discussion	frequency polygon
references	normal distribution
tables	skew
figures	"blind" review

REFERENCES

Anastasi A: Psychological Testing, ed. 3. New York, Macmillan Co., 1968

American Psychological Association: Publications Manual of the American Psychological Association, ed. 3. Washington, DC, American Psychological Association, 1983

Ayres AJ: A form used to evaluate the work behavior of patients. American Journal of Occupational Therapy 8:73, 1954

Belson WA: The Design and Understanding of Survey Questions. Aldershot, England, Gower Publishing, 1981

Berg IA: Response bias and personality: The deviation hypothesis. Journal of Psychology 40:61, 1955

Berg IA: Deviant responses and deviant people: The formulation of the deviation hypothesis. Journal of Counseling Psychology 4:154, 1957

Berg IA: The unimportance of test item content. In Bass BM, Berg IA (eds): Objective Approaches to Personality Assessment. Princeton, NJ, Van Nostrand, 1959

Berg IA: Measuring deviant behavior by means of deviant response sets. In Berg IA, Bass BM (eds): Conformity and Deviation. New York, Harper, 1961

Best JW: Research in Education, ed. 4. Englewood Cliffs, NJ, Prentice Hall, 1981

Bradburn NM, Sudman S: Improving Interview Method and Questionnaire Design. San Francisco, Jossey-Bass, 1979

Brown EM, Van der Bogert M: Prevocational motor skill inventory. American Journal of Occupational Therapy 7:153, 1953

Bunge M: Scientific Research. I: The Search for System. Studies in the Foundations, Methodology and Philosophy of Science, vol 3. New York, Springer-Verlag, 1967

208

Buros OK: Test in Print. Highland Park, NJ, Gryphon Press, 1974

Buros OK: The Eighth Mental Measurements Yearbook. Highland Park, NJ, Gryphon Press, 1978

Campbell DT: Stereotypes and the perception of group differences. American Psychologist 32:817, 1967

Campbell DT, Stanley JC: Experimental and Quasi-Experimental Designs for Research. Boston, Houghton Mifflin, 1963

Carlsmith JM, Ellsworth PC, Aronson E: Methods of Research in Social Psychology. Reading, MA, Addison-Wesley, 1976

Carr LG: Sexrole items and acquiescence. American Sociological Review 36:287, 1971

Cook TD, Campbell DT: Quasi-Experimentation: Design and Analysis Issues for Field Settings. Chicago, Rand McNally, 1979

Cozby PC: Methods in Behavioral Research. Palo Alto, CA, Mayfield Publishing, 1977

Crowne DP, Marlowe D: The Approval Motive: Studies in Evaluative Dependence. New York, Wiley, 1964

Currier DP: Elements of Research in Physical Therapy, ed. 2. Baltimore, MD, Williams & Wilkins, 1984

DeLameter J: Response-effects of question content. In Dijkstra W, van der Zouwen J (eds): Response Behavior in the Survey-Interview. Oxford, England, Academic Press, 1982

Dixon WJ (ed): BMDP Statistical Software, 1981 edition. Los Angeles, University of California Press, 1981

Downs CW, Smeyak GP, Martin E: Professional Interviewing. New York, Harper & Row, 1980

Ehrlich JS, Reisman D: Age and authority in the interview. Public Opinion Quarterly 25:39, 1961

Ethridge DA, McSweeney M: Research in Occupational Therapy. Dubuque, IA, Kendall/Hunt Publishing, 1971

Festinger L, Carlsmith JM: Cognitive consequences of forced compliance. Journal of Abnormal and Social Psychology 58:203, 1959

Finn J: Multivariance: Univariate and Multivariate Analysis of Variance, Covariance, Regression, and Repeated Measures. Version 6. A Fortran IV program. Chicago, National Educational Resources, 1978

Hagenaars JA, Heinen TG: Effects of role-independent interviewer characteristics on responses. In Dijkstra W, Van der Zouven J: Response Behavior in the Survey-Interview. Oxford, England, Academic Press, 1982

Hochstim JR, Renne KS: Reliability of response in a sociomedical population study. Public Opinion Quarterly 35:69, 1971

Hull CH, Nie NH: SPSS: Update 7-9. New York, McGraw-Hill, 1981

Isshiki KR: Small Business Computers. Englewood Cliffs, NJ, Prentice-Hall, 1982

Kerlinger F: Foundations of Behavioral Research. New York, Holt, Rinehart and Winston, 1965

Koller E: Personal communication, 1960. In Richardson SA, Dohrenwend BS, Klein D: Interviewing: Its Forms and Functions. New York, Basic Books, 1965

Kuhn TS: The Structure of Scientific Revolutions. Chicago, University of Chicago Press, 1962

Labaw PJ: Advanced Questionnaire Design. Cambridge, MA, Abt Books, 1980

Linton M: A Simplified Style Manual for the Preparation of Journal Articles in Psychology, Social Sciences, Education, and Literature. New York, Appleton-Century-Crofts, 1972

McClave JT, Benson PG: Statistics for Business and Economics, ed. 3. San Francisco, Dellen Publishing, 1985

Masters WH, Johnson VE: Human Sexual Response. New York, Little, 1966

Michels E: Research and human rights, 2. Physical Therapy 56:546, 1976

Molenaar HJ: Response-effects of "formal" characteristics of questions. In Dijkstra W, van der Zouwen J (eds): Response Behavior in the Survey-Interview. Oxford, England, Academic Press, 1982

Nie NH, Hull CH, Jenkins JG, Steinbrenner K, Brent DH: SPSS: Statistical Package for the Social Sciences, ed. 2. New York, McGraw Hill, 1975

Orlich DC: Designing Sensible Surveys. Pleasantville, NY, Redgrave Publishing, 1978

Orne M: Demand characteristics and the concept of quasi-controls. In Rosenthal R, Rosnow R (eds): Artifacts in Behavioral Research, New York, Academic Press, 1969

Osgood CE, Suci GJ, Tannenbaum PH: The Measurement of Meaning. Urbana, IL, University of Illinois Press, 1957

Payne S: The Art of Asking Questions. Princeton, NJ, Princeton Press, 1951

Polit DF, Hungler BP: Nursing Research: Principles and Methods, ed. 3. Philadelphia, J B Lippincott, 1987

Reed KL: Models of Practice in Occupational Therapy. Baltimore, Williams & Wilkins, 1984

Reynolds PD: A Primer of Theory Construction. Indianapolis, Bobbs-Merrill, 1971

Richardson SA, Dohrenwend BS, Klein D: Interviewing: Its Forms and Functions. New York, Basic Books, 1965

Rosenthal R, Lawson R: A longitudinal study of the effects of experimenter bias on the operant learning of laboratory rats. Journal of Psychiatric Research 2:61, 1964

Roy SC, Roberts SL: Theory Construction in Nursing: An Adaptation Model. Englewood Cliffs, NJ, Prentice-Hall, 1981

SAS Institute Inc. SAS User's Guide: Basics, 1982 edition. Cary, NC, SAS Institute, 1982

SAS Institute Inc. SAS User's Guide: Statistics, 1982 edition. Cary, NC, SAS Institute, 1982

Smith SL: Physical capacities evaluation. In Hopkins H, Smith H: Willard & Speckman's Occupational Therapy, ed. 5. Philadelphia, J B Lippincott, 1978

Spector PE: Research Designs. Beverly Hills, CA, Sage Publications, 1984

SPSS Inc. SPSSX: User's Guide. New York, McGraw-Hill, 1983

Trombly CA, Scott AD: Occupational Therapy for Physical Dysfunctions. Baltimore, MA, Williams & Wilkins, 1977

Turabian KL: A Manual for Writers of Term Papers, Theses, and Dissertations, ed. 4. Chicago, University of Chicago Press, 1973

Weick KE: Systematic observational methods. In Lindzey G, Aronson E (eds): The Handbook of Social Psychology, vol. 2, ed. 2. Reading, MA, Addison-Wesley, 1968

GLOSSARY

abstract—Short summary of research generally appearing at beginning of research report. Collections may appear in research journals and in indexes to be found in library.

acquiescence bias—tendency on part of some respondents on research questionnaires to respond affirmatively to all items.

active independent variable—independent variable to be manipulated by investigator (e.g., level of drug dosage).

alpha level—level (determined by investigator) of strength of statistical evidence necessary to declare results of study statistically significant.

alternative hypothesis (also known as experimental hypothesis)—hypothesis stating relationship between variables that will be tested indirectly by research study. (The null hypothesis is tested directly.) Rejection of null hypothesis results in acceptance of alternative hypothesis.

analysis of covariance (ANCOVA)—statistical procedure that allows investigator to control for intervening variables that are not of interest to study but may affect values obtained for dependent measures.

analysis of variance (ANOVA)—statistical procedure that allows means of more than two groups to be compared simultaneously while maintaining control of probability of Type I error.

applications software—computer languages and programs that allow user to direct computer in analysis of data, handling of files, etc.

applied research—research that is intended to address specific practical problem.

ARIMA (autoregressive integrated moving average)—statistical techniques to be applied for analysis of interrupted time series data.

arithmetic-logic unit—part of computer hardware in central processing unit in which actual data analysis is conducted.

array—arrangement of study data in which obtained scores are ordered sequentially from lowest to highest.

assembly language—lowest-level computer language, in which instructions are given in complex alphanumerical codes. Intermediate between high-level languages and machine code.

attribute independent variable—independent variable whose categories are subject characteristics such as age or gender that cannot be manipulated or assigned by investigator.

bar charts—pictorial presentation primarily employed with nominal data.

basic research—research conducted to broaden knowledge but without particular practical goal or application in mind.

beta—statistical term referring to probability of making Type II error.

bias—distortion introduced into research data. May be introduced by experimenter, data collection instrumentation, subjects, or analytical procedures.

"blind" review—process in which evaluators of grant applications or submissions for publication in journals are kept ignorant of author's name and affiliation. Intended to reduce subjectivity in review process.

"blind" techniques—techniques intended to reduce occurrence of experimental bias from expectancy effects or demand characteristics. The experimenter in actual contact with subjects is kept ignorant of subjects' category and of experimental hypotheses. Experimenters cannot communicate information that they do not possess.

case study (report)—type of research in which single situation or individual is studied in depth.

cathode ray tubes (CRTs)—television-like monitors frequently seen on microcomputers.

central processing unit (CPU)—part of computer hardware containing arithmetic-logic and control units.

central tendency—descriptive statistics calculated to describe "average" or most representative score of data set. Includes mean, median, and mode.

checklists—possible format for use on written questionnaires. Subjects read list of items and indicate with check-mark those that are applicable.

chi square test—statistical technique applied to nominal data that compares observed frequency of phenomenon with expected frequency. The three basic forms are simple chi square, contingency chi square, and "goodness of fit" test.

class boundaries—points at two ends of classes in frequency distribution determined by investigator as impossible (unattainable) values falling halfway between actual top value of one class and actual lowest value of subsequent class.

class mark—midpoint of class in frequency distribution. Calculated by adding class boundaries and dividing by two.

closed questions—questions on either questionnaires or interviews in which responses are constrained into given format by investigator.

cluster sampling—type of probability sampling in which several successive random samples are chosen from increasingly smaller populations.

coefficient of determination (r²)—statistic calculated in conjunction with linear regression or correlation. Indicates amount of variability in measures that is accounted for by their relationship.

cohort—group of individuals moving through some process as a group, such as classmates in school.

concept coding—translation of raw data into form appropriate for data analysis based on underlying ideas expressed in data.

concurrent validity—type of test validity. A test is considered to possess concurrent validity if it correlates with valid test measuring same construct.

consistency effect—sequence effect that may be observed in interviews or written questionnaires. Subjects' earlier answers make certain issues salient in their minds, and subsequent answers are chosen to be consistent with earlier responses.

construct validity—type of validity of concern in design of study and of data collection instruments. Theoretical constructs must be thoroughly conceptualized and measured in study.

content validity—type of test validity that concerns extent to which content of test measures phenomenon of interest.

continuous variable—variable whose measures do not fall into neat, separable units. Continuous measures cannot be precisely measured.

contrast effect—sequence effect in interview in which earlier responses create contrast with later responses.

control—one of characteristics of "true experiments."

control group—group of subjects that serves as comparison group for experimental group. Most frequently left untreated, but (when practical or ethical constraints apply) may be group that receives different treatment from true experimental group.

control unit—part of computer hardware in central processing unit.

convenience sampling—type of nonprobability sampling. Subjects for sample are chosen because they are conveniently available to investigator.

correlated groups t *test*—one of group of parametric tests designed to compare means either of two groups matched on some characteristic or of two scores obtained under different treatment conditions by same individuals.

correlation—several statistical procedures that measure extent of covariation between two sets of data. The Spearman Correlation is applied to ordinal data, Pearson Product-Moment Correlation to ratio or interval data.

criterion-related validity—type of test validity concerned with extent to which test correlates with other known measures of phenomenon. Includes concurrent and predictive validity.

criterion variable—type of dependent variable in which measured level of variable is established as level indicating acceptable performance.

critical value—obtained value for inferential statistical procedures that has probability of occurrence (given true null hypothesis) equal to alpha level.

cumulative frequency—column in frequency distribution that indicates summative frequency of class and all classes below.

cyclical variability—component of time series analysis. Regular variability that has cycle longer than one year.

debriefing—meeting at end of study (especially studies containing deception) at which investigator explains purpose of study.

deception—misrepresention of true purposes or hypotheses of study to those who are to participate in it. Intended to reduce demand characteristics.

degrees of freedom—statistical term indicating number of measures in data that are free to vary. Often employed in conjunction with probability tables to determine critical value of statistic.

demand characteristics—conditions set up by experimenter that provide subjects with clues about anticipated experimental behaviors.

dependent variables—data measures in research study. Believed to depend for their value on subjects' level of independent variable.

descriptive research—type of non-experimental research. Includes: (1) survey research, (2) observational research, (3) time series research, (4) secondary analysis, (5) historical research, (6) evaluation research, and (7) methodological research.

deviation bias—response bias leading subjects to choose most extreme response independent of item content.

deviation scores—distance of each raw data measure from mean of distribution. Always sum to zero.

discrete variable—measure in which units are neat, separable units such as number of chairs.

discussion—final narrative section of research report in which results are explained and conclusions are drawn.

"downstream periscope"—theory of perception in which all perceptions are biased by attitudes, beliefs, and previous learning before ever reaching consciousness.

evaluation research—research intended to determine effectiveness of program or intervention such as legislation.

expectancy effects—response bias in which subjects unconsciously attempt to tailor responses to what they perceive as experimenter's expectations.

experiment—research endeavor characterized by three characteristics: control, manipulation, and randomization.

experimental bias—*see* bias.

experimenter bias—distortion introduced into research data by behaviors, expectations, or attitudes of experimenters.

ex post facto research—non-experimental research that measures variables in attempt to establish relationships between them.

external validity—applicability of results of research study in other settings.

field experiment—research conducted in "real world."

formative evaluation research—descriptive research conducted at beginning of program or intervention to determine form program or intervention should take.

frame of reference—basic level of model of scientific development. Involves scientists' knowledge and attitudes affecting their perceptions of world.

frequency polygon—pictorial representation of ratio data in research report.

"guggles"—one-syllable sounds emitted by interviewer to indicate to respondent that he or she wishes to speak.

Guttman scale—format for questionnaire response. Also known as cumulative scale because agreement with each higher level of response indicates agreement with all levels below chosen response.

halo effects—two types of response bias in which one overwhelming characteristic influences responses to whole subject area (either one extremely positive trait increases positivity to entire area or one extremely negative trait lowers all ratings of area).

hardware—1. Mechanical components of computer. 2. Mechanical data collection instruments.

histogram—graphic form resembling bar charts. Pictorial representation of data.

historical research—research that examines historical documents and artifacts.

homogeneity of variance—underlying assumption of parametric statistical tests. Assumes that variances of parent populations of sample groups are comparable.

hypothesis—statement presenting suspected relationship between variables to be tested in research. (*See* alternative hypothesis *and* null hypothesis).

hysteresis—characteristic of mechanical data collection instrumentation in which readings from instrument are dependent on direction on scale in which readings are taken.

independent groups t *test*—one of group of parametric tests that compares means of separate, independent groups on data measures.

independent variable—phenomenon of interest in research study. Effects of different levels of independent variable are believed to differ on dependent (outcome) measures.

informed consent—agreement of subject to participate in study based on full communication of potential risks by experimenter.

input device—part of computer hardware that accepts information into computer system.

instrument effects—experimental bias introduced by data collection instruments.

internal validity—consistency of relationship of variables within research study that precludes explanations for research results other than experimental hypotheses.

inter-rater reliability—consistency of observation between observers in research study.

interrupted time series—experimental manipulation introduced into time series measures to determine effect of intervention.

interval scale—measurement scale in which measurement points have equal inter-measure intervals but which has no real zero point.

intervening variables—variables that may appear between independent and dependent measure but that are not of interest to research study.

interviews—method of data collection that involves direct contact between individuals. May be conducted in person or by telephone.

irregular variability—component of time series data. Variability that cannot be accounted for by trend, seasonal variability, or cyclical variability.

keypunch—device used in preparation of data cards for early form of computer input device.

Kruskal-Wallis Test—nonparametric equivalent of analysis of variance. Allows for simultaneous comparison of more than two groups while controlling probability of Type I error.

laboratory experiment—research conducted in controlled environment (as opposed to field experiment).

Likert scale—format for questionnaire in which subjects indicate degree of agreement along continuum from agree to disagree.

linearity—characteristic of mechanical data collection instruments.

linear regression—statistical procedure that determines extent to which knowledge of values of one variable allow for accurate prediction of values of another variable.

manipulation—one of characteristics of true experiments. Experimenter actively changes levels of independent variable.

matrix—format for questionnaires that involves expanded checklist. Instead of merely checking response, subject has several response choices for each question.

mean—most commonly employed measure of central tendency. Also known as "average."

median—measure of central tendency. Point in data array at which 50% of data points fall below and 50% fall above.

methodological research—research intended to improve data collection procedures and instruments.

methods—section of research report that indicates procedures, equipment, and subjects.

mode—measure of central tendency. Most commonly occurring score(s).

Model—representation of reality based on relationship between variables. Between theory and frame of reference in scientific development.

multiple choice—format for closed questions in questionnaire. Subject must choose from several options.

multiple regression—statistical technique employed to determine accuracy with which scores for variable may be predicted from knowledge of more than one other variable.

negativity bias—response bias in which subject responds negatively to all questionnaire or interview items.

nominal scale—measurement scale in which measures consist of categories of data rather than numerical measures.

non-equivalent control groups—group used in type of quasi-experimental research in which, because of lack of randomization, control groups cannot be assumed to be similar to treatment groups.

non-experiment—research that does not involve any manipulation on part of researcher.

non-parametric tests—less powerful class of statistical techniques that do not rest on any underlying assumptions about parent populations of sample groups.

nonprobability sampling—less desirable group of sampling techniques in which subject selection is based on subjective decisions of investigator rather than any probability scheme.

non-schedule interview—standardized interview in which interviewer is free to vary question wording and order.

normal distribution—symmetrical distribution on which parametric statistics are based.

null hypothesis—hypothesis tested directly through use of inferential statistics. States that no difference exists between experimental groups or that experimental treatment was not effective.

observational research—non-experimental research in which investigators record observations of subject behaviors.

observer bias—subjectivity introduced through process of observation.

open-ended questions—interview questions that do not constrain subject to any particular format of response.

operational definition—definition based on techniques (or operations) needed to measure variable.

ordinal scale—measurement scale in which data represent rank orderings of measures.

output device—part of computer hardware that communicates results of computer's processing of data.

paradigm—system that organizes theories into coherent, comprehensive overview of discipline.

parametric tests—powerful inferential statistical techniques to be employed only when underlying assumptions of homogeneity of variance and normal distribution are satisfied.

Pearson Product-Moment Correlation—statistical technique that measures extent of covariation between two measures.

pie charts—pictorial representation of nominal data.

placebo—inert substance given to subjects who believe they are receiving "real" experimental treatment. Used to counter expectancy effects.

post hoc fallacy—incorrect belief that because two variables occur sequentially, earlier variable caused later variable.

power—ability of statistical technique to find effect that does exist.

predictive validity—type of test validity. Test correlates with tests of same characteristic taken at later time.

probability sampling—superior form of choosing samples for research. Each element in population has known probability of being selected for sample.

prospective studies—type of ex post facto research. Postulates relationship between variables before collection of data.

proxy pre-tests—measures employed before treatment that are not to be employed after treatment. Should correlate highly with post-test measures.

purposive sampling—type of nonprobability sampling in which investigator chooses subjects on the basis of some subjective criterion.

quasi-experiment—research that is lacking either randomization or control (characteristics of "true" experiments). Often conducted in field settings.

questionnaires—written data collection instruments.

quota sampling—nonprobability method of sampling in which sample is stratified and then strata are filled through nonprobability methods.

random assignment—assignment of chosen subjects to experimental condition on the basis of random assignment procedures.

range—1. Measure of variability obtained by subtracting lowest obtained score from highest obtained score. 2. Breadth of measurement range of mechanical data collection equipment.

rapport effect—positive sequence effect in interview. Increased exposure to interviewer generally increases respondents' level of comfort and rapport, resulting in less defensive and more candid responses later in interview.

ratio scale—measurement scale in which intervals between measurement points are equal and there is true zero point.

reference group effect—sequence effect in interviews and questionnaires in which earlier questions increase salience of attitudes and beliefs of subject's reference group. Subsequent responses are more likely to be in direction of reference group's norms.

references—bibliographical listing at end of research report in which cited literature is catalogued.

region of rejection—area of distribution of statistical scores that contains percentage of scores determined by alpha level.

regression-discontinuity studies—type of research in which assignment to treatment condition is based on pre-test scores.

relative frequency—part of frequency distribution in which frequency of each class is presented as proportion of entire data set.

reliability—stability or trustworthiness of measure.

replication—repeating study to determine if results will appear again.

research ethics—basic principles of good research that protect subjects from harm.

response bias—tendency on part of subjects to respond in patterned set.

results—portion of research report in which statistical analyses of data are reported.

retrospective studies—ex post facto studies that measure variable changes that have already occurred.

routing—ordering of questions in interview or questionnaire so as to help avoid chances of sequence effects.

saliency effect—sequence effect in questionnaire or interview in which responses to earlier questions have sensitized subject to particular topic.

sample—smaller subset of population, chosen to represent population in research. Can be chosen by probability or nonprobability methods.

schedule interview—type of standardized interview in which interviewer is not allowed to vary wording or order of questions from set schedule.

secondary analysis—type of research in which data collected by others is subjected to re-conceptualization and analysis.

seasonal variability—component of time series data that occurs cyclically within period of one year.

semantic differential—type of format for questionnaires. Employs pairs of adjectives with scale between.

sequence effects—potential biases determined by order in which questions appear in either questionnaires or interviews.

simple random sampling—type of probability sampling in which each element of population has equal probability of being selected into sample

single sample t *test*—one of family of parametric tests that compares mean of single sample to known population mean.

skew—departure of distribution from symmetry in which one end of distribution ends in elongated "tail."

snowball sampling—type of nonprobability sampling in which subjects are asked to recruit new subjects for study.

social desirability bias—possible response bias on questionnaires in which respondent responds to items in socially desirable direction.

software—languages and programming that direct computer in data processing.

Spearman correlation—statistical technique that measures extent of covariation in two sets of ordinal data.

split-half reliability—technique for assessing test reliability in which answers to items are divided into two equal groups and scores are calculated on groups and compared.

standard deviation—most frequently employed measure of variability.

standardized interview—type of interview in which same data is elicited from all subjects.

statistical conclusion validity—type of validity based on appropriate use of statistical procedures.

status survey—type of survey research that seeks to collect data on currently existing conditions.

stepwise regression—type of multiple regression statistical technique in which predictor variables are added into equation incrementally.

storage unit—"memory" of computer system.

stratified sampling—type of probability sampling in which there are recognizable groups (or strata) within population that are to be matched in sample. The requirements for numbers of subjects in each strata are identified, then probability sampling techniques are employed for actual subject selection.

summative evaluation research—research conducted at end of program or intervention intended to evaluate effectiveness of program.

survey research—research that employs questionnaires to collect data.

symbolic language—high-level computer programming language such as FORTRAN.

systematic sampling—method of sampling in which every case element is chosen for inclusion.

systems software—basic command languages that are used internally within computer; not generally used by outside users.

tables—summaries of statistical information usually appearing in results section of research report.

test-retest reliability—stability of test determined by administering test, waiting interval, re-administering test, and correlating two scores.

test validity—"accuracy" of test. Includes content validity, criterion-related validity, and construct validity.

theory—systematizing of information and facts in discipline into set of hypothesized relationships. Considered to occupy place between model and paradigm in development of scientific discipline.

time series analysis—series of measures collected over period of time without intervention or experimental manipulation that are analyzed into trend, seasonal variability, cyclical variability, and irregular variability.

trend—component of time series data. Represents long-term gradual change.

t *tests*—group of parametric statistical techniques that compare means of groups to determine whether groups are significantly different.

Type I error—claiming that effect exists when in fact it does not. Controlled by setting of alpha level.

Type II error—failing to detect effect that exists.

unstandardized interview—interview in which data collected from subjects differs between subjects in study.

validity—"accuracy" of study or data collection instrument. Includes internal validity, statistical conclusion validity, construct validity, external validity, content validity, and criterion-related validity.

variance—measure of variability. Equal to square of standard deviation.

variables—measures in study that do not have fixed values.

Wilcoxon rank sum text—nonparametric equivalent to independent groups *t* test.

Wilcoxon signed rank test—nonparametric equivalent to *t* test for single samples and correlated groups.

word coding—inferior method of transposing interview data into analyzable form solely on basis of appearance of certain words in protocol.

□□□□□□□□
INDEX

Page numbers in italics indicate figures; page numbers followed by t indicate tabular material.